20 different sports and 150 of the hardest races in history

THE WORLD'S
Toughest
ENDURANCE RACES

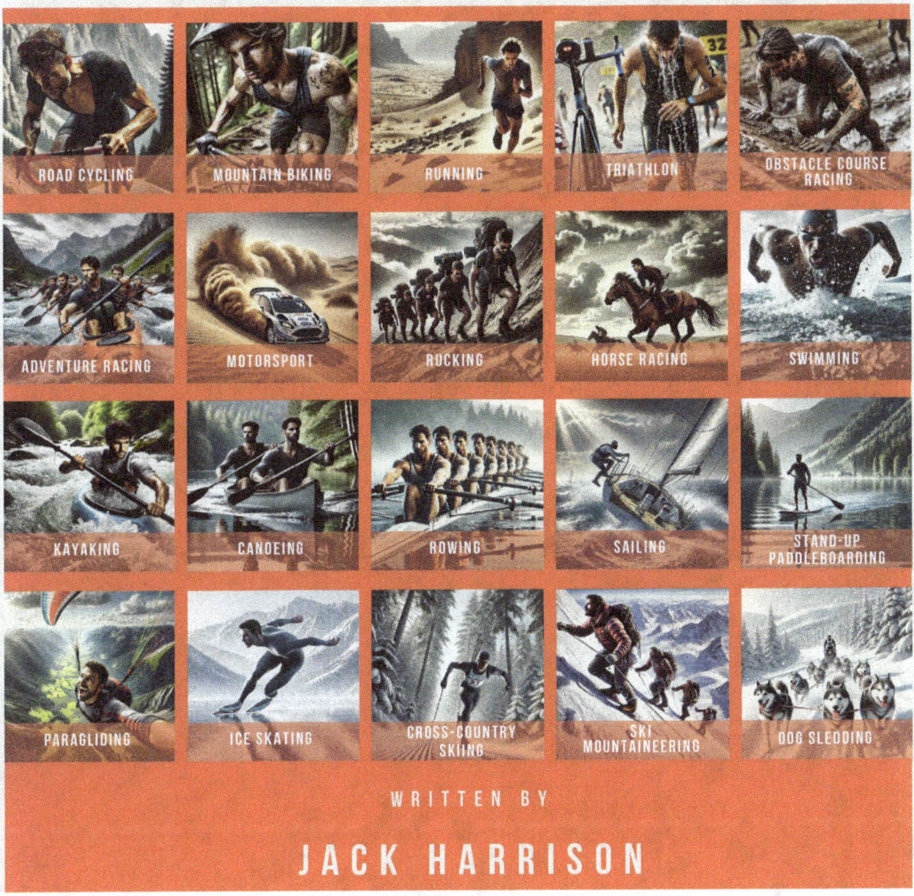

ROAD CYCLING

MOUNTAIN BIKING

RUNNING

TRIATHLON

OBSTACLE COURSE RACING

ADVENTURE RACING

MOTORSPORT

RUCKING

HORSE RACING

SWIMMING

KAYAKING

CANOEING

ROWING

SAILING

STAND-UP PADDLEBOARDING

PARAGLIDING

ICE SKATING

CROSS-COUNTRY SKIING

SKI MOUNTAINEERING

DOG SLEDDING

WRITTEN BY

JACK HARRISON

THE WORLD'S *Toughest* ENDURANCE RACES

20 different sports and 150 of the hardest races in history

For those seeking inspiration to push their physical limits far beyond what they imagined possible, or for those who find enjoyment in reading about the challenges others have overcome to complete the world's toughest endurance races.

JACK HARRISON

COPYRIGHT

All rights reserved. No part of "The Worlds Toughest Endurance Races" may be reproduced, stored in a retrieval system, or transmitted in any form or by any means - electronic, mechanical, photocopying, recording, or otherwise without the prior written permission of the publisher, except in the case of brief quotations embodied in critical articles and reviews. This book is a work of non-fiction based on the author, Jack Harrison's, experiences, research, and insights into the world of endurance racing. The events, locales, and conversations are drawn from the author's personal encounters and a wide range of secondary sources. While extensive efforts have been made to ensure the accuracy of information contained in this publication, the publisher and author assume no responsibility for errors, inaccuracies, or omissions. Any slights of people, places, or organisations are unintentional.

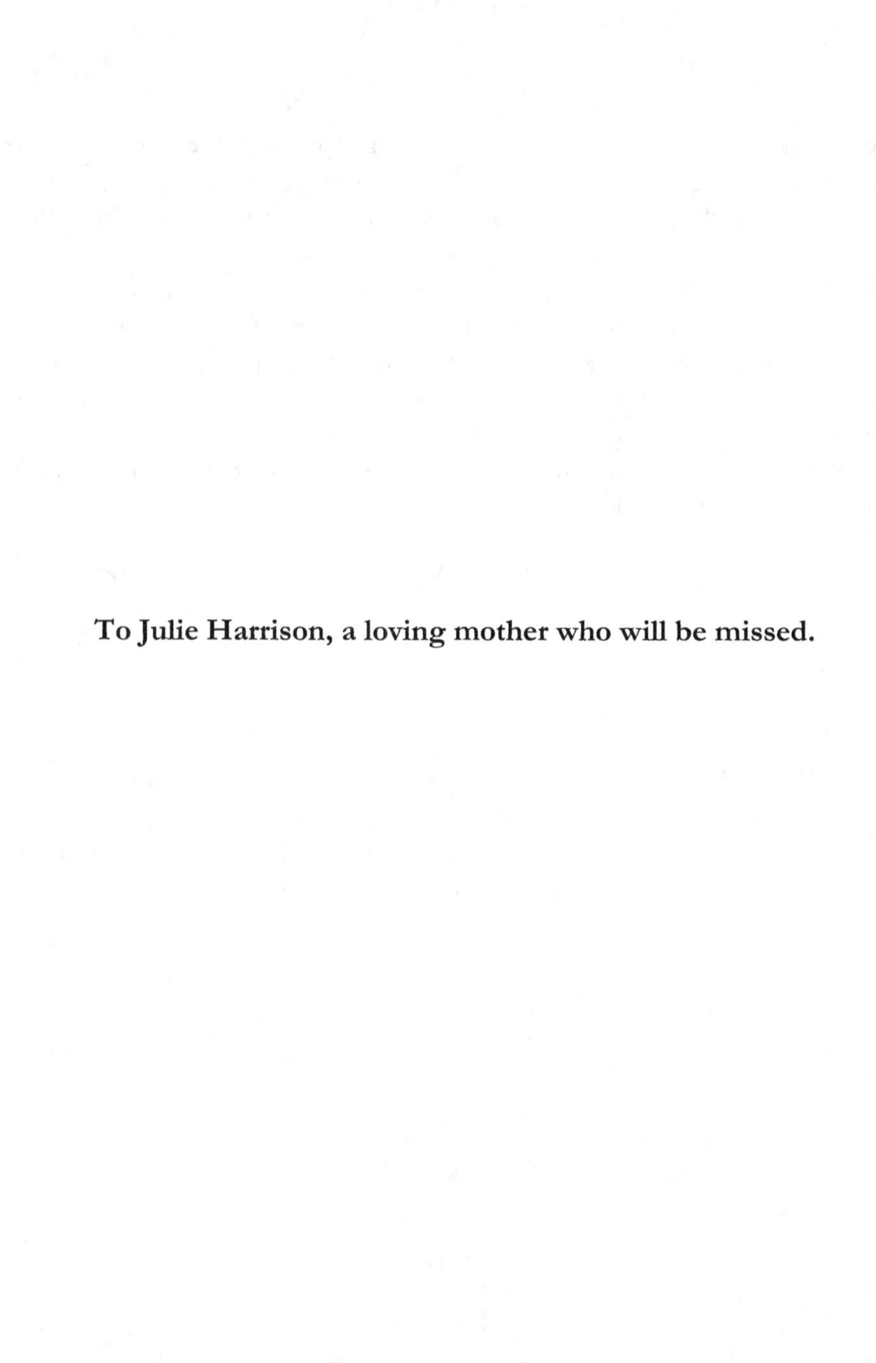

To Julie Harrison, a loving mother who will be missed.

TABLE OF CONTENTS

INTRODUCTION 10

CHAPTER 1 - LAND SPORTS 11

ROAD CYCLING 12

Trans Am Bike Race 14

Race Across America 15

NorthCape 4000 16

Transcontinental Race 17

Cent Cols Challenge 18

Trans Pyrenees Race 19

London-Edinburgh-London (LEL) 20

Paris-Brest-Paris (PBP) 21

Race Across Switzerland (RAS) 22

Haute Route Alps 23

MOUNTAIN BIKING 24

The Tour Divide 26

Silk Road Mountain Race 27

Arizona Trail 800 28

Atlas Mountain Race 29

The Trans Pyr 30

Colorado Trail Race 31

Cape Epic 32

Iditarod Trail 350 Invitational 33

The Yak Attack 34

Andes Pacifico 35

RUNNING 36

Self-Transcendence Race 38

Yukon Arctic Ultra 39

The Spine Race 40

Moab 240 41

Tor Des Géants 42

Grand To Grand Ultra 43

Marathon Des Sables 44

Spartathlon 45

Jungle Ultra 46

Badwater 135 47

Ultra Trail Du Mont Blanc 48

Hardrock Hundred 49

Barkley Marathon 50

Western States Endurance Run 51

TRIATHLON 52

The Epic5 Classic 54

Bretzel Ultra Quintuple Triathlon 55

Enduroman 56

The Ultraman Canada 57

The Ultraman Australia 58

Austria Extreme Triathlon 59

Norseman 60

Swissman 61

OBSTACLE COURSE RACING.. 62

Spartan Death Race.. 64
Spartan Agoge.. 65
World Toughest Mudder.. 66
Iron Viking... 67

ADVENTURE RACING.. 68

Patagonian Expedition Race.. 70
Expedition Alaska... 71
Adventure Racing World Championship.. 72
Legend Expedition Race.. 73
Primal Quest... 74
Coast-To-Coast New Zealand.. 75
Wilderness Traverse.. 76
Red Bull Defiance... 77

MOTORSPORT.. 78

Around The World In 80 Days Rally.. 80
Iron Butt Rally.. 81
Peking To Paris... 82
Dakar Rally... 83
Africa Eco Race.. 84
East African Safari Rally.. 85
24 Hours Of Le Mans.. 86
Irondog... 87
24 Hours Of Daytona.. 88
Cains Quest.. 89
Baja 1000.. 90
Mille Miglia.. 91

RUCKING... 92

Nijmegen Marches.. 94
GORUCK Selection.. 95
Cateran Yomp... 96
Winter Death Race.. 97
Bataan Memorial Death March.. 98
Tough Ruck Boston... 99

HORSE RACING... 100

Mongol Derby... 102
Shahzada Memorial Endurance Test.. 103
The Tevis Cup... 104

CHAPTER 2 - AIR SPORTS... 105

PARAGLIDING..106

Icarus Trophy..108
Red Bull X-Alps.. 109
X-Pyr.. 110
Vercofly...111
Transdromoise..112
Bornes To Fly.. 113
X-Scotia Hike and Fly... 114

CHAPTER 3 - SNOW SPORTS...115

ICE SKATING...116

Weissensee...118
Baikal Wild Ice Grand Marathon...119
Finland Ice Marathon...120
Skate The Lake...121

CROSS COUNTRY SKIING...122

Nordenskiöldsloppet...124
Arctic Circle Ski Race...125
Canadian Ski Marathon...126
Vasaloppet...127
La Transjurassienne...128
Marcialonga...129
Finlandia-Hiihto...130
Tartu Ski Marathon...131
American Birkenbeiner...132
Birkebeinerrennet...133
König Ludwig Lauf...134
Engadin Skimarathon...135

DOG SLEDDING...136

Iditarod Trail...138
Finnmarksløpet...139
Kobuk 440...140
Femundløpet...141
Canadian Challenge...142
La Grande Odyssée...143

SKI MOUNTAINEERING...144

Pierra Menta...146
Tour du Rutor...147
Andorra Skimo 10...148
The Grand Traverse...149
Patrouille Des Glaciers...150
Trofeo Mezzalama...151
Adamello Ski Raid...152
Sellaronda Ski Marathon...153
Altitoy-Ternua...154

CHAPTER 4 - WATER SPORTS...155

SWIMMING...156

20 Bridges Swim...158
Capri-Napoli...159
Lake Zurich Swim...160
Port to Pub...161
Vidösternsimmet...162
The Rottnest Channel Swim...163

KAYAKING...164

Yukon 1000...166

Race To Alaska..167
Missouri River 340...168
The WaterTribe Everglades Challenge..169
Texas Water Safari...170
Massive Murray Paddle...171

CANOEING..172

La Ruta Maya Belize River Challenge...174
Devizes To Westminster International Canoe Race (DW)....................175
AuSable River Canoe Marathon...176
Adirondack Canoe Classic...177
Dusi Canoe Marathon...178
The Hawkesbury Canoe Classic..179

SAILING...180

Volvo Ocean Race..182
Clipper Round the World Yacht Race..183
Golden Globe Race...184
Vendee Globe..185
Transat Jacques Vabre..186
Transatlantic Race...187
Transpacific Yacht Race..188
Rolex Fastnet Race...189
Bermuda Race...190
Sydney to Hobart Yacht Race..191

ROWING...192

Talisker Atlantic Challenge..194
Great Pacific Race..195
GB Row Challenge..196
Tour Du Léman à l'Aviron..197
Ringvaart Regatta..198

STAND-UP PADDLEBOARDING...199

Yukon River Quest..201
SUP 11 City Tour..202
The Crossing For Cystic Fibrosis...203
Molokai 2 Oahu...204

CONCLUSION..205

AUTHOR...206

INTRODUCTION

I'll be honest, this book was never meant to be a book. I'm certainly no author, and I didn't set out with the intention of writing one. What began as a simple collection of notes about races I wanted to do in the future gradually turned into something more. Over time, I realized that there are many people out there, like me, who love pushing their limits. That's when it hit me, why not share that with others who thrive off the same challenges. And so, this book was born.

Throughout my journey, I've been fortunate to meet hundreds of people with the same mentality. Those who want to push their limits and see just how far their bodies can go. For us, it's about more than just finishing a race. It's about wearing each accomplishment like an internal badge of honor, knowing that we've gone the distance. If you're reading this and nodding along, then I hope this book serves as a guide, a roadmap for you to discover new challenges, test your physical and mental limits, and perhaps plan your next big adventure.

This book is for those who are curious, like me, about what the human body can achieve when truly tested. Maybe you're here because you're drawn to the thrill of endurance racing or searching for new, daunting races to tackle. Or perhaps you're simply fascinated by the extraordinary feats of endurance these races represent. Whatever your reason, I invite you to explore these pages and dive into the realm of the world's toughest endurance races.

But this book is more than just a list of gruelling races, it's a tribute to the athletes who push their absolute limits and the race organizers who make these events possible year after year. As you read, I hope you gain a deeper appreciation for those who have crossed the finish line and feel inspired to one day stand at the starting line yourself.

Endurance racing has come a long way since I started writing this book. I remember when running a marathon was seen as the ultimate test of long-distance stamina. Now, it's not uncommon to meet people who regularly compete in ultra-marathons or tackle extreme challenges across various sports. The distances are getting longer, the times more demanding, and the boundaries of human capability continue to be pushed year after year.

So, without further ado, let me introduce you to what I believe are the world's toughest endurance races. My hope is that these pages will inspire you to lace up your shoes, hop on your bike, or dive into the pool with renewed motivation and excitement.

Enjoy.

CHAPTER 1 – LAND SPORTS

In this chapter, I will delve into the realm of land-based sports, which form the foundation of many of the world's toughest endurance races. While some of these races may occasionally feature other elements, such as kayaking in adventure races or swimming legs in triathlons, the foundation of these events is still faced on solid terrain. Land sports are, in many respects, the purest form of human competition. Running, for instance, is one of the simplest and most fundamental activities, requiring nothing more than the human body and a pair of shoes. This simplicity gives land-based sports a timeless quality, linking us to the earliest days of human competition.

It's no surprise that these types of sports are likely among the oldest forms of organized competition. As a result, this chapter features more events than those that incorporate water, air-based elements and snow. The accessibility of land-based sports has also allowed them to maintain their popularity throughout history. From casual recreational runs to elite marathons and ultra-endurance races, the appeal of testing one's physical and mental strength on the ground is universally felt. These sports have developed into some of the most gruelling endurance tests imaginable, constantly evolving to meet the desires of athletes looking for new challenges. Whether running, cycling, or hiking, the commonality is that they can create the ultimate test of stamina and resilience. In this chapter, I will explore what I consider to be the world's most difficult land-based endurance races. Whether you're a seasoned athlete or a novice, these races symbolize the pinnacle of human strength and endurance. Let's begin our journey with road cycling.

ROAD CYCLING

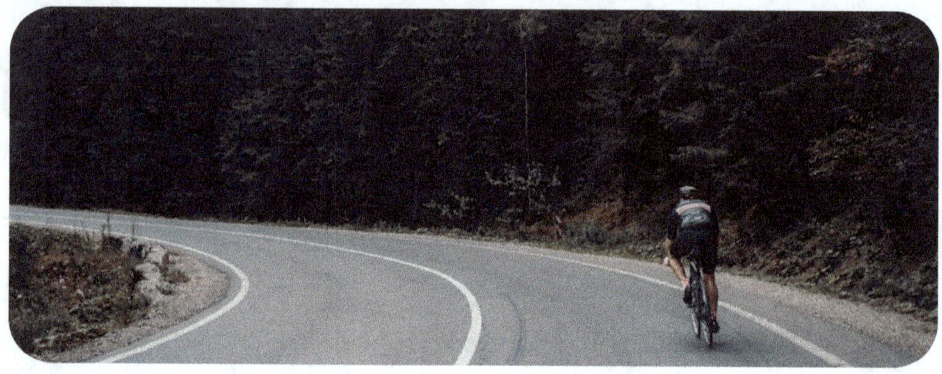

Road cycling is categorised as a competitive sport where cyclists race on paved roads. These races can vary widely in format, from one-day classics to multi-stage tours that span several days or even weeks. In road racing, competitors navigate courses that often include a mix of undulating terrain and challenging climbs. During these races, riders must deal with factors like weather, road conditions, elevation and altitude.

Road cycling's history dates back to the late 19th century. The sport began to gain prominence with the first organised races in Europe, with one of the earliest major events being the Paris-Roubaix, first held in 1896, which remains one of the most prestigious one-day races today. The Tour de France later came into existence in 1903 and is perhaps the most iconic road cycling event. Over time, road cycling has evolved with advancements in technology, such as lighter bicycles and more efficient gear systems, and the thus the sport has expanded globally, becoming a major component of the international sports calendar.

The concept of long endurance races in road cycling became formalized in the early 20th century with the introduction of multi-stage races that challenged riders' stamina over multiple days. The Giro d'Italia, first held in 1909, stands as a prominent early example, featuring a demanding route that spans thousands of kilometres across varied terrain. Another key event is the Vuelta a España, which began in 1935. These pioneering events set the standard for long-distance road cycling, and their structure laid the foundation for the modern endurance races we see today.

Road cycling races have become increasingly demanding due to advancements in technology, evolving race formats, and rising competitive standards. Modern races often feature more challenging courses with steeper climbs, longer distances, and more technical sections. The development of high-performance bicycles, such as aerodynamic frames and advanced gear systems, has enabled cyclists to achieve higher speeds and tackle more difficult terrain. Additionally, race organizers have introduced new formats and stages, including time trials, mountain stages, and mixed-terrain routes, adding more layers of complexity. The growing level of competition, with more professional and elite cyclists participating, has also intensified the racing environment, pushing riders to continuously adapt and refine their training and tactics. This evolution reflects a broader trend towards more challenging road cycling events and who knows what races there might be in the future.

When selecting what I consider the toughest road cycling races in the world, I focused primarily on two key factors: distance and elevation gain. Longer distances mean more hours in the saddle, and over time, fatigue inevitably sets in. Elevation gain adds another layer of difficulty, especially in unsupported races where participants carry a significant amount of gear. Environmental factors, such as weather conditions and road surfaces, also play a major role, forcing cyclists to adapt to shifts in temperature, wind, and terrain. This often requires them to carry additional clothing and equipment as well. The races detailed in this chapter are among the most challenging I could find, many of which have been running for over a decade and have rightly earned their reputation as some of the toughest in the sport.

Without further ado, lets delve into the toughest road cycling races in the world.

TRANS AM BIKE RACE

- **Location**.. United States
- **Time of year**................................... June
- **Approximate distance**.................. 6920km (4300 miles)
- **Average time to finish**................. 16 - 30 days
- **Average number of entries**.......... 100 - 150 participants
- **Average cost to enter**................... $200 - $300
- **Year it started**............................. 2014
- **Support offered**........................... Unsupported

The Trans AM Bike Race (TABR) is one of the premier unsupported ultra-distance cycling events that spans the width of the United States from coast to coast. First starting in 2014, the race quickly found a reputation for being one of the most gruelling challenges within the ultra-cycling realm. The route they use was inspired by the iconic TransAmerica Trail, which has been a favoured route for long-distance cyclists for nearly 50 years. Each year, cyclists from around the world test their limits, relying solely on their own resources to navigate the route and complete the race.

The course of the Trans AM Bike Race stretches approximately 6920km (4300 miles) from Astoria, Oregon to Yorktown, Virginia. This journey traverses ten states, crossing the Rocky Mountains, the Great Plains, and the Appalachian Mountains, offering incredible views and some naughty elevation gain! The race is renowned for its steep climbs, unpredictable weather conditions and the endurance required to ride continuously with minimal sleep. Cyclists must navigate through some of the most remote areas of the US with limited access to amenities, making planning and resourcefulness crucial to the race. The unsupported nature of the race adds another layer of difficulty, as participants cannot receive outside assistance and must carry their own gear and provisions.

Prospective participants need to register through the official race website, where they can find detailed information on race rules, requirements, and route details. The entry fee typically ranges from $200 - $300, reflecting the race's minimalist, self-supported ethos.

You can find further information about the TABR on their official website: transambikerace.com.

RACE ACROSS AMERICA

- **Location**.................................... United States
- **Time of year**................................ June
- **Approximate distance**................. 4800km (3000 miles)
- **Average time to finish**................ 6 – 12 days
- **Average number of entries**.......... 200 – 300 participants
- **Average cost to enter**................... $2000 – $5000
- **Year it started**............................ 1982
- **Support offered**........................... Supported

The Race Across America (RAAM) is potentially the most prestigious and well-known ultra-distance road cycling race in the world. It was first held in 1982 and has since become a fixture in the global cycling endurance events calendar. The race is a true test of endurance and has grown in stature ever since it's beginning to attract elite cyclists and ambitious amateurs from all around the world. Unlike some of the other stage races, the RAAM is a continuous race from start to finish, which means the clock never stops. Competitors must manage their own strategy for rest and recovery, making it as much a mental challenge as a physical one.

Starting in Oceanside, California, and finishing in Annapolis, Maryland, the RAAM covers approximately 4800km (3000 miles) across 12 states. The route traverses the deserts of Arizona, the Rocky Mountains of Colorado, and the Great Plains, before tackling the Appalachian Mountains, presenting riders with extreme changes in elevation and weather. The course's total vertical climb exceeds 170,000 feet, which is nothing to be sniffed at. Riders can look forward to facing upwards of 22 hours per day in the saddle and this relentless demand makes the RAAM perhaps the ultimate test in endurance cycling.

To enter the RAAM, participants must meet certain qualification criteria. This can include completing RAAM-qualified events or demonstrating experience in other ultra-endurance races. The race is open to solo riders and teams, which can range from two to eight cyclists. Teams can participate in a relay format which allows for a faster time and an easier race. Personal support crews are mandatory for all participants.

You can find further information about the RAAM on their official website: www.raceacrossamerica.org

NORTHCAPE 4000

- Location................................... Europe
- Time of year............................. July
- Approximate distance................. 4000km (2485 miles)
- Average time to finish................. 10 - 21 days
- Average number of entries.......... 100 - 150 participants
- Average cost to enter.................. $300 - $700
- Year it started........................... 2017
- Support offered......................... Unsupported

The NorthCape 4000 is one of the most adventurous events Europe has to offer, challenging participants to cycle over 4000km (2485 miles) from Italy to the northernmost point of Europe, the North Cape in Norway.

The route covers a variety of terrains and landscapes, from the alpine climbs of Austria, the forests of Finland and the fjords of Norway. What makes the race particularly challenging is not just the distance, but the variety of weather conditions encountered along the way. Riders face unpredictable weather that can range from scorching heat to near-freezing temperatures which can cause problems particularly in an unsupported race.

To enter the NorthCape 4000, participants need to register on the official event website where they can also find detailed information about the race rules, entry fees, and required equipment. The race is open to solo riders and occasionally pairs. Entries are usually limited to ensure the quality and safety of the experience of all participants.

You can find further details about the NorthCape 4000 on their official website: www.northcape4000.com.

TRANSCONTINENTAL RACE

- **Location**... Europe
- **Time of year**.................................... July/ August
- **Approximate distance**................. 4000km (2485 miles)
- **Average time to finish**................. 7 - 15 days
- **Average number of entries**.......... 200 – 300 participants
- **Average cost to enter**.................... $200 - $400
- **Year it started**............................. 2013
- **Support offered**........................... Unsupported

The Transcontinental Race (TCR) is a self-supported race across Europe, known for the vast distance it covers. It was first held in 2013 and founded by Mike Hall, a legend in the ultra-endurance cycling community. The TCR challenges riders to traverse the European continent with predefined checkpoints while choosing their own paths in between. Therefore, this race is not just a test of physical endurance but also of riders navigation skills and self-sufficiency.

The TCR course varies each year but typically spans approximately 4000km (2485 miles), starting from one corner of Europe and finishing in another. It also often incorporates several of Europe's iconic climbs and regions. The varied terrain, which can include high mountain passes and long stretches of flatlands, tests the cyclists' ability to adapt their riding to different conditions and to make sure their route navigation is good enough that they know what they're going to encounter.

Entering the Transcontinental Race requires participants to apply through an entry process that often includes a questionnaire designed to assess their experience and readiness for the race. It generally opens for entries in the autumn for the following year's edition, and spots are highly sought after and often filled quickly.

You can find further information about the TCR on their official website: www.transcontinental.cc.

CENT COLS CHALLENGE

- **Location**..................................... Europe
- **Time of year**.............................. August/ September
- **Approximate distance**................. 2000km (1242 miles)
- **Average time to finish**................ 10 days
- **Average number of entries**.......... 30 – 40 participants
- **Average cost to enter**.................. $3000 - $4500
- **Year it started**............................ 2009
- **Support offered**........................... Supported

The Cent Cols Challenge is an extraordinary cycling event that tests the endurance of passionate cyclists who aim to complete one hundred mountain passes (cols) in just ten days. The idea was created by Phil Deeker in 2009 as part of his personal quest to ride one thousand cols in one summer. It has since evolved into a series of events held in various mountainous regions of Europe, including the Alps, Pyrenees, and Dolomites. The challenge attracts riders from around the world who are drawn not only by the physical challenge but also by the landscape Europe has on offer.

The Cent Cols Challenge is renowned for its demanding nature, primarily due to the sheer number of high-altitude ascents which are packed into a relatively short period. Each edition of the challenge covers different routes but always involves climbing around 20,000 meters over 2000 kilometres. The routes are carefully designed to include some of the most iconic and lesser-known cols, providing a thorough test of climbing ability and endurance. Weather conditions can greatly increase the difficulty, as participants often face the unpredictability of mountain weather, including cold, rain, or extreme sun. The physical demands, combined with the mental challenge of enduring ten consecutive days of intense cycling, make the Cent Cols Challenge a formidable endeavour to any cyclist.

Those interested in participating must apply through the official Cent Cols Challenge website, where they can also find detailed information about the various editions of the race, including route details, logistical arrangements, and entry fees. The challenge is supported, with the organization providing logistical support, meals, and guidance, but the riding is independent.

You can find details about the Cent Cols Challenge on their official website: www.centcolschallenge.com

TRANS PYRENEES RACE

- **Location**..................................... France & Spain
- **Time of year**................................ October
- **Approximate distance**................. 1500km (932 miles)
- **Average time to finish**................. 6 – 10 days
- **Average number of entries**.......... 100 participants
- **Average cost to enter**.................. $200 – $700
- **Year it started**............................. 2018
- **Support offered**........................... Unsupported

The Trans Pyrenees Race is a relatively new cycling event that has been launched by Lost Dot, the same organization behind the Transcontinental Race. This event was introduced to offer a similarly gruelling challenge but within the iconic terrain of the Pyrenees mountains. The race requires participants to navigate a course that spans the full length of the Pyrenees from the Atlantic to the Mediterranean, while being self-supported and navigating some of the most challenging climbs Europe.

The Trans Pyrenees course is a traverse of one of Europe's most famous mountain ranges. Stretching approximately 1500km (932 miles), the route includes significant elevation gain, often exceeding 40,000 meters across the entirety of the race. This route not only challenges riders with its endless climbs but also with its descents, which require an abundance of technical skill. The terrain varies from well-paved roads to potentially rough, less-travelled paths that can vary in technicality dramatically depending on the weather conditions.

Entry into the Trans Pyrenees Race requires cyclists to demonstrate a proven track record in endurance cycling, given the extreme demands of the event. The registration process typically involves an application where riders must detail their cycling experience and readiness, this is undoubtably why the race is capped at a small number of participants to maintain safety and support standards, making entry competitive.

You can find more info about the Trans Pyrenees race on their official website: https://www.lostdot.cc/race-brand/trans-pyrenees

LONDON-EDINBURGH-LONDON (LEL)

- **Location**.. United Kingdom
- **Time of year**............................... August (every four years)
- **Approximate distance**.................. 1400km (870 miles)
- **Average time to finish**................. 80 – 120 hours
- **Average number of entries**........... 1000 – 1200 participants
- **Average cost to enter**................... $150 – $250
- **Year it started**.............................. 1980
- **Support offered**............................ Supported

This race was first held in 1980 as a response to the growing popularity of endurance cycling. The event, organized by the Audax UK cycling club, follows a 1,400km route between London and Edinburgh, with a return leg to London. The race is part of a tradition of long-distance cycling events that include other notable events like Paris-Roubaix and the Paris-Brest-Paris. Over the years, LEL has grown into one of the most challenging and respected ultra-distance cycling events globally.

The LEL course is renowned for its difficulty due to its sheer length, diverse terrain, and unpredictable weather conditions. The route traverses a range of landscapes, including the rolling hills of the English countryside, the undulating terrain of the Scottish Highlands. Cyclists face numerous challenges, including significant elevation changes that test their climbing abilities and varying road surfaces to test their bike handling skills. The course is separated by several checkpoints where riders can rest, resupply, and receive mechanical support, but the vast distances between these checkpoints mean that cyclists must be self-reliant and well-prepared for long stretches of riding to meet strict time limits for each stage.

Entering the LEL requires participants to meet specific qualifications and strict criteria. Prospective riders must have completed at least two qualifying brevets, or long-distance rides, including one of 300km or more, within the year leading up to the event. The entry fee covers logistical support, including access to checkpoints, mechanical assistance, and safety measures throughout the race. Securing a spot in the race often involves a lottery or a selection process to ensure all participants are adequately prepared.

You can find more information about the LEL on their official website:
https://londonedinburghlondon.com/

PARIS-BREST-PARIS (PBP)

- **Location**.. France
- **Time of year**................................. August
- **Approximate distance**................. 1200km (745 miles)
- **Average time to finish**................. 45 – 90 hours
- **Average number of entries**........... 6000 participants
- **Average cost to enter**................... $200 – $300
- **Year it started**............................. 1891
- **Support offered**............................ Unsupported

Paris-Brest-Paris (PBP) is one of the oldest and most renowned long-distance cycling events in the world. First held in 1891 as a professional race, then converted into an amateur event in 1931, the PBP sadly only runs every four years and is organized by the Audax Club Parisien. Over the decades, PBP has maintained its allure and challenge, drawing cyclists from all around the globe who come to test their limits.

The Paris-Brest-Paris course extends over approximately 1200km (745 miles) and requires riders to complete the route within a 90 hour time limit, although faster time limits are set for different categories of riders. The route takes participants from the Parisian suburbs to the city of Brest on the Atlantic coast and back, traversing a varied landscape that includes rolling hills and flat pastoral lands. Riders must be prepared for all weather conditions, and the event often includes riding through both day and night which adds a layer of complexity with clothing and nutrition to stay on form for such a long amount of time.

Entry into Paris-Brest-Paris requires qualification through a series of events in the years leading up. Cyclists must complete a series of official rides of 200, 300, 400, and 600km organized by recognized organisations worldwide. These qualifying events are designed to prepare riders for the PBP and ensure they can handle the challenge. Detailed information about the qualification process, registration details, and more can be found on the official PBP website.

You can find more information about the PBP on their official website:

www.paris-brest-paris.org

RACE ACROSS SWITZERLAND (RAS)

- **Location**.................................... Switzerland
- **Time of year**............................... July
- **Approximate distance**................. 1000km (620 miles)
- **Average time to finish**................ 70 – 100 hours
- **Average number of entries**.......... 100 – 150 participants
- **Average cost to enter**................... $200 – $300
- **Year it started**............................. 2007
- **Support offered**........................... Supported

The Race Across Switzerland is a ultra-endurance event known for its challenging course across the Swiss Alps. It has quickly become one of the most demanding cycling races in Europe, attracting elite and amateur cyclists who seek to push their limits. The race is organized by a dedicated team with a passion for ultra-distance cycling and a deep respect for the beauty of Switzerland. As an integral part of the ultra-cycling calendar, RAS offers cyclists a unique opportunity to experience the country's breathtaking landscapes while enduring a physically and mentally taxing competition. Over the years, it has gained a reputation for its rigorous demands and the exceptional resilience required to complete it, reflecting the growing global interest.

The route takes cyclists through the heart of the Swiss Alps, including several high-altitude mountain passes such as the Furka, Grimsel, and Susten Passes. These climbs present significant elevation gains and require exceptional climbing skills and physical endurance. The course's difficulty is compounded by Switzerland's variable weather conditions, which can range from sunny and warm to cold and rainy, often within the same day. Riders face a combination of steep ascents, technical descents, and fast, flat sections.

Prospective riders typically need to demonstrate prior experience in long-distance cycling, often by completing qualifying races or brevets of significant distances, such as 300km or more. This requirement ensures that all entrants possess the necessary endurance to handle the RAS. The entry fee covers various race logistics, including route support, checkpoint facilities, and safety measures. Spots can be limited, and entries may be subject to a lottery or selection process.

You can find details about the Race Across Switzerland on their website: https://raceacrossseries.com/en/race-across-suisse/

HAUTE ROUTE ALPS

- **Location**.................................... France & Switzerland
- **Time of year**............................. August
- **Approximate distance**................. 800km (497 miles)
- **Average time to finish**................. 7 days
- **Average number of entries**........... 400 – 500 participants
- **Average cost to enter**................... $1500 – $2200
- **Year it started**............................ 2011
- **Support offered**........................... Supported

The Haute Route Alps is a multi-day event known as the highest and toughest cyclosportive in the world. First launched in 2011, the Haute Route has expanded to include several iterations in iconic cycling locations around the globe. However, the Alps edition remains the flagship event. This race attracts amateur cyclists who want to experience what it is like to ride a professional tour under similar conditions. The event spans over seven consecutive days and covers some of the most famous climbs in cycling, offering participants a blend of competitive racing and spectacular landscapes.

The Haute Route Alps course covers over 800km (497 miles) and features more than 20,000 meters of climbing. It is designed to mimic the stage profiles of Grand Tour racing, incorporating legendary Alpine climbs such as the Col du Galibier and Alpe d'Huez. Each stage presents its own challenges, from long climbs and technical descents to potential weather changes that can include heat or sudden Alpine storms. The cumulative fatigue over a week of high-altitude riding tests the physical and mental limits of participants, making it one of the most difficult amateur cycling events in the world.

Entry into the Haute Route Alps is open to any amateur cyclist looking for a challenge. Participants can enter as individuals or as part of a team. The registration process involves choosing a package that can include full logistical support, such as accommodations, meals, race support, and additional services.

You can find more details about the Haute Route Alps on their official website: www.hauteroute.org

MOUNTAIN BIKING

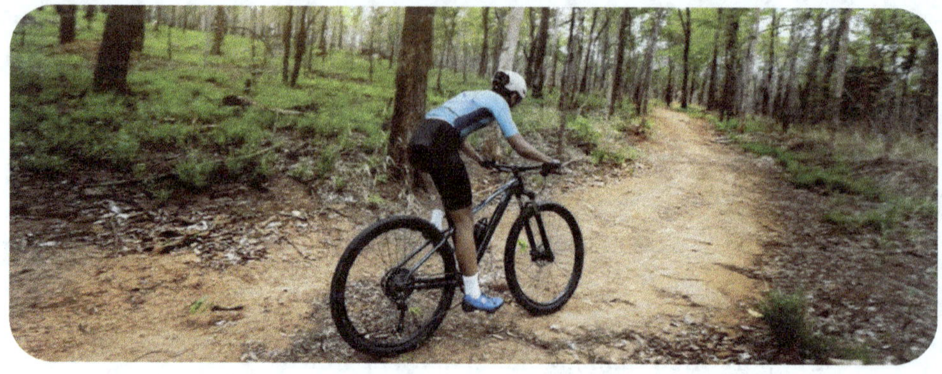

Mountain biking is an exhilarating and physically demanding sport where cyclists navigate off-road terrain on bikes designed to handle rough trails and obstacles. In cross-country races, competitors cover a series of laps on a circuit that includes climbs, descents, and technical features, with the goal of completing the course in the shortest amount of time. However, in ultra-endurance mountain bike races, routes are often designed with the goal of getting from point A to point B in the shortest time possible, sometimes even allowing for undefined paths. Many of the long-distance races mentioned in this chapter also require participants to carry all their own gear, as bikepacking has become a popular approach in long-distance cycling events.

Mountain biking as a distinct sport began to take shape in the 1970s, primarily in California, where enthusiasts adapted traditional bicycles for off-road use. The sport's origins are often traced to pioneers like Gary Fisher, Tom Ritchey, and Joe Breeze, who modified bikes with sturdy frames, wide tires, and suspension systems to tackle trails in the Marin County area. The first mountain bike race is credited to the Repack Downhill race held in 1976, which marked the beginning of competitive mountain biking. The 1980s saw the establishment of formal organizations and the first official mountain biking events, including the National Off-Road Bicycle Association (NORBA) in 1983. The sport quickly gained popularity, leading to the development of a global racing scene, with key events such as the UCI Mountain Bike World Cup and the introduction of mountain biking as an Olympic sport in 1996.

Long mountain biking endurance races began to gain prominence in the 1980s and 1990s, as the sport matured, and riders sought to test their stamina over extended distances and challenging conditions. One of the earliest and most notable long endurance events is the Leadville Trail 100, which was first held in 1983. This race, set in the high-altitude terrain of Leadville, Colorado, covers 100 miles of trail with significant elevation changes, demanding both physical endurance and technical skill.

Another significant early endurance event is the Dirty Kanza (now known as Unbound Gravel), which began in 2006 and features a gruelling 200-mile gravel race. These early events set benchmarks for mountain bike endurance racing.

Mountain biking races have become increasingly challenging as the sport has evolved and technology has advanced. Modern races often feature more demanding courses with steeper climbs, more technical descents, and complex terrain, reflecting the growing advancements of bike design and rider skills. Advances in technology, such as more effective suspension systems, lighter frames, and high-performance tires, have enabled riders to tackle more difficult and varied courses. Additionally, the rise of ultra-endurance events, such as 24-hour races and multi-day stage races, has pushed the boundaries of physical endurance.

When identifying the toughest mountain bike races in the world, I believe, as with road cycling, that the key factors pushing participants to their limits are distance and elevation gain. However, other elements come into play as well. Unsupported races, where riders must rely solely on the gear they can carry, significantly increase the level of difficulty. Additionally, weather conditions can greatly impact a rider's speed and performance - anyone who has cycled through thick mud or snow knows how challenging it can be. It's this combination of factors that has earned the following races a spot on the list of the toughest mountain bike events in the world. So, let's dive in and explore what's on offer.

THE TOUR DIVIDE

- **Location**.. United States & Canada
- **Time of year**............................... June
- **Approximate distance**.................. 4418km (2745 miles)
- **Average time to finish**.................. 15 – 25 days
- **Average number of entries**.......... 150 – 200 participants
- **Average cost to enter**................... Free
- **Year it started**.............................. 1999
- **Support offered**............................ Unsupported

The Tour Divide is one of the most challenging ultra-endurance mountain bike races in the world, tracing the spine of the Rocky Mountains along the Great Divide Mountain Bike Route (GDMBR). The Tour Divide runs from Banff, Alberta, Canada, to Antelope Wells, New Mexico, USA, inviting cyclists to take on the landscapes of North America in a test of stamina and navigation. This race is renowned for its self-supported ethos and it's $0 entry fee, this means it requires a a high level of preparation from its participants.

The Tour Divide covers approximately 4418km (2745 miles) making it one of the longest off road cycling routes in the world. The route features over 200,000 feet of elevation gain, traversing a mix of dirt roads, forest paths, and mountain bike trails. Riders face extreme weather conditions, varying from snowy mountain passes in Canada to the desert heat of New Mexico, along with the challenges posed by remote wilderness areas where wildlife encounters are common. The route's length and the physical demand of continuous self-supported cycling, combined with the logistical challenge of managing supplies over weeks of riding, contribute to its reputation as a formidable endeavour which is not to be taken lightly.

Entry into the Tour Divide does not follow a conventional registration process due to its self-supported and informal nature. Riders who wish to participate typically show up at the start line in Banff on the designated start day in June and race. There is no official entry fee, but participants must be fully self-sufficient, carrying all necessary equipment and managing their own logistics throughout the race.

You can find more information about the Tour Divide on their official website: http://tourdivide.org/

SILK ROAD MOUNTAIN RACE

- **Location**... Kyrgyzstan
- **Time of year**................................. August
- **Approximate distance**................. 1700km (1056 miles)
- **Average time to finish**................. 7 – 14 days
- **Average number of entries**.......... 50 – 100 participants
- **Average cost to enter**.................... $300 – $800
- **Year it started**.............................. 2018
- **Support offered**............................ Unsupported

The Silk Mountain Race is a bikepacking event that traverses the historic Silk Road. Established relatively recently, this race seeks to blend endurance cycling with a journey through the landscapes that once hosted ancient trade routes. Participants in the Silk Mountain Race experience not only a physical challenge but also a historical expedition, riding through regions rich in tradition.

The Silk Mountain Race course covers several countries, following parts of the old Silk Road that connect Europe and Asia. The exact route can vary, but it typically includes high mountain passes, arid deserts, and remote wilderness areas. The difficulty of the race is worsened by the extreme climates along the route, from freezing mountain temperatures to blistering desert heat and the varying road conditions, which can range from paved highways to unmaintained trails. This race not only tests physical endurance but also demands significant navigational skills and self-sufficiency, as services and support are sparse along much of the route.

Interested cyclists should have experience in long-distance bikepacking and be prepared for the self-supported nature of the race. Prospective participants can find entry details, race rules, and equipment recommendations on the race's official website. Registration usually opens several months in advance, with various categories available to accommodate solo riders and teams.

You can find more info about the Silk Mountain race on their official website:
https://www.silkroadmountainrace.com/

ARIZONA TRAIL 800

- **Location**.................................... Arizona (United States)
- **Time of year**................................ October
- **Approximate distance**.................. 1287km (800 miles)
- **Average time to finish**................. 7 – 14 days
- **Average number of entries**.......... 60 participants
- **Average cost to enter**................... $100 – $200
- **Year it started**............................. 2006
- **Support offered**........................... Unsupported

The AZT800, also known as the Arizona Trail 800, is an extreme mountain bike race that challenges riders to traverse the entire length of the Arizona Trail from the borders of Mexico to Utah. This race is a test of endurance, skill, and self-sufficiency, designed for only the most experienced of bikepackers. The event, which started gaining popularity in the early 2010s, has quickly become a bucket-list race for ultra-endurance mountain bikers, drawing participants who are eager to tackle one of the toughest trails in North America.

The AZT800 covers terrain that includes steep mountain passes, long desert stretches, and rocky canyons. The trail is notorious for its technical difficulty, requiring riders to navigate sharp rocks and other challenging obstacles. Elevation changes are drastic and frequent, testing the climbing and descending of every rider. Additionally, the race occurs in a region known for its extreme weather conditions, where temperatures can soar during the day and plummet at night, adding an extra layer of difficulty. The remote nature of much of the trail means that riders must be entirely self-reliant, carrying all necessary supplies for repairs and rest.

Entering the race typically opens a few months before the event and is handled online. Participants are expected to have significant experience in long-distance bikepacking and must be equipped with gear that can withstand the harsh conditions of the Arizona Trail. Due to the extreme nature of the race, the number of entries is often limited.

You can find more details about the AZT800 on their official website:
https://azt300-800.com

ATLAS MOUNTAIN RACE

- **Location**................................... Morocco
- **Time of year**.............................. February
- **Approximate distance**................. 1200km (745 miles)
- **Average time to finish**................. 5 – 10 days
- **Average number of entries**.......... 100 – 150 participants
- **Average cost to enter**................... $300 – $400
- **Year it started**............................. 2020
- **Support offered**.......................... Unsupported

The Atlas Mountain Race is a relatively new yet rapidly growing fixture in the bikepacking race calendar. First launched in 2020, the event takes place in Morocco and invites participants to navigate a route through the Atlas Mountains. This self-supported bikepacking race draws cyclists who are eager to test their endurance across North Africa's most demanding and scenic trails.

 Spanning over 1200km, the course of the Atlas Mountain Race winds through the remote areas of the Atlas Mountains, featuring elevations that can exceed 2000 meters. The route is characterized by a mix of rocky paths, dirt roads, and occasional stretches of sand, making both navigation and physical progress challenging. Riders face extreme variations in temperature, from cold mountain nights to hot days under the desert sun. This range of conditions, combined with the need to be self-sufficient (carrying all necessary food, water, and equipment), makes the Atlas Mountain Race a true test of a cyclist's resilience, technical skills, and mental toughness.

Entry into the Atlas Mountain Race requires cyclists to have a solid background in endurance cycling, particularly in self-supported events. Interested participants must register online, where they can also find detailed information about the race requirements, equipment guidelines, and tips for preparation. The race typically opens for entries several months in advance, and spots are limited to maintain a manageable scale for safety.

You can find more info about the Atlas Mountain race on their official website: www.atlasmountainrace.cc.

THE TRANS PYR

- **Location**.. Spain & France
- **Time of year**............................... June
- **Approximate distance**................. 800km (500 miles)
- **Average time to finish**................ 7 – 12 days
- **Average number of entries**.......... 200 – 300 participants
- **Average cost to enter**.................. $800 – $2000
- **Year it started**............................ 2010
- **Support offered**........................... Supported

The Trans Pyr is a challenging mountain bike race that tests cyclists across the harsh terrain of the Pyrenees. This mountain range forms a natural border between France and Spain and makes for great mountain biking too. The event was designed to offer an extreme test of endurance and technical skill, pushing participants to their limits as they traverse east to west, from the Mediterranean to the Atlantic. The race combines demanding physical challenges with incredible scenery, and as such has attracted an international field of experienced riders since its beginning.

Spanning approximately 800km (500 miles), the Trans Pyr course is renowned for its gruelling profile, featuring steep ascents, rapid descents, and technical single-track sections through some of the most remote parts of the Pyrenees. Participants face a cumulative elevation gain that can exceed 20,000 meters. The varied terrain, from rocky paths and forest trails to high mountain passes tests even the most seasoned of cyclist. Weather conditions in the mountains can be unpredictable, adding another layer of difficulty as riders cope with potential extremes from scorching heat to chilling winds and rain.

Entry into the Trans Pyr is highly competitive, catering primarily to experienced mountain bikers due to the technical and physically demanding nature of the course.

You can find more information about the Trans Pyr on their official website: https://www.transpyr.com/

COLORADO TRAIL RACE

- **Location**.................................... Colorado (United States)
- **Time of year**................................ July
- **Approximate distance**................. 800km (500 miles)
- **Average time to finish**................ 4 – 7 days
- **Average number of entries**.......... 70 – 100 participants
- **Average cost to enter**.................. Free
- **Year it started**............................ 2007
- **Support offered**........................... Unsupported

The Colorado Trail Race (CTR) is an ultra-endurance mountain bike race that takes riders through some of the most scenic and challenging landscapes in the United States. The race, which started in 2007, is held annually and traverses the entire length of the Colorado Trail, stretching from Denver to Durango. The CTR has quickly become a hallmark event in the bikepacking community, drawing cyclists looking to test their limits against the rugged backdrop of the Colorado Rockies. Unlike many organized races, the CTR is a grassroots event, emphasizing self-reliance.

The course of the Colorado Trail Race covers over 500miles and features a staggering 70,000ft of elevation gain. The trail includes steep climbs, technical descents, and high-altitude passes that reach up to 13,000ft. Riders face a variety of terrains, from rocky mountain paths to forest trails, each presenting its own set of challenges. Weather conditions can also vary dramatically along the route, from intense sunshine and heat to sudden thunderstorms and even snow, depending on the elevation and time of year.

Entering the Colorado Trail Race does not involve a formal registration process or fee. Instead, riders are expected to show up at the designated start time and place, typically announced on the race's informal website and through community forums. Participants must be fully self-supported, carrying all necessary gear for navigation, camping, and repairs. There is no official support, and riders must adhere to strict leave-no-trace principles to minimize their impact on the trail.

You can find more info about the Colorado trail race on their official website:
https://jwookieone.com/2024-colorado-trail-race/

CAPE EPIC

- **Location**...................................... Colorado (United States)
- **Time of year**............................... July
- **Approximate distance**................. 800km (500 miles)
- **Average time to finish**................ 4 – 7 days
- **Average number of entries**.......... 70 – 100 participants
- **Average cost to enter**.................. Free
- **Year it started**............................ 2007
- **Support offered**........................... Unsupported

The Colorado Trail Race (CTR) is an ultra-endurance mountain bike race that takes riders through some of the most scenic and challenging landscapes in the United States. The race, which started in 2007, is held annually and traverses the entire length of the Colorado Trail, stretching from Denver to Durango. The CTR has quickly become a hallmark event in the bikepacking community, drawing cyclists looking to test their limits against the rugged backdrop of the Colorado Rockies. Unlike many organized races, the CTR is a grassroots event, emphasizing self-reliance.

The course of the Colorado Trail Race covers over 500miles and features a staggering 70,000ft of elevation gain. The trail includes steep climbs, technical descents, and high-altitude passes that reach up to 13,000ft. Riders face a variety of terrains, from rocky mountain paths to forest trails, each presenting its own set of challenges. Weather conditions can also vary dramatically along the route, from intense sunshine and heat to sudden thunderstorms and even snow, depending on the elevation and time of year.

Entering the Colorado Trail Race does not involve a formal registration process or fee. Instead, riders are expected to show up at the designated start time and place, typically announced on the race's informal website and through community forums. Participants must be fully self-supported, carrying all necessary gear for navigation, camping, and repairs. There is no official support, and riders must adhere to strict leave-no-trace principles to minimize their impact on the trail.

You can find more info about the Colorado trail race on their official website:
https://jwookieone.com/2024-colorado-trail-race/

IDITAROD TRAIL 350 INVITATIONAL

- **Location**.. Alaska (United States)
- **Time of year**............................... February
- **Approximate distance**................. 560km (350 miles)
- **Average time to finish**................. 3 – 6 days
- **Average number of entries**.......... 50 – 100 participants
- **Average cost to enter**................... $1000 – $1500
- **Year it started**............................. 2007
- **Support offered**........................... Unsupported

The Iditarod Trail 350 Invitational is an extreme endurance race that tests participant survival skills and physical limits in the harsh Alaskan wilderness. Originating in 2000, the race is a shorter version of the more extensive Iditarod Trail Invitational, which continues to Nome, following the legendary Iditarod sled dog race route. Designed for the toughest outdoor adventurers, the race includes categories for bikers, runners, and skiers. It not only draws seasoned ultra-endurance athletes but also those seeking to experience one of the most challenging and remote trails under extreme winter conditions.

Spanning 560km (350 miles) from Knik to McGrath, the course goes through deep forests, frozen rivers and mountain ranges. The difficulty of the Iditarod Trail 350 is amplified by the brutal Alaskan winter weather, with temperatures often dropping far below zero. Coupled with unpredictable snow conditions and potential whiteouts, the weather condition in this race must be some of the most challenging of any endurance race. Navigation can also be an issue n these conditions and the isolation of the trail means that self-sufficiency is crucial. Participants must carry mandatory survival gear and be prepared to tackle any emergency on their own, making this race not just a physical challenge but a significant mental ordeal as well.

Entry into the Iditarod Trail 350 Invitational is highly competitive, with potential participants required to demonstrate proven experience in winter survival skills and ultra-long-distance racing. The race typically limits its entries to ensure safety and manageability. Those interested in participating must apply well in advance and often need to qualify through other similar endurance events.

You can find more details about the Iditarod Trail 350 on their official website: https://itialaska.com/

THE YAK ATTACK

- **Location**... Nepal
- **Time of year**.................................... October/ November
- **Approximate distance**................. 500km (310 miles)
- **Average time to finish**................. 7 – 10 days
- **Average number of entries**.......... 50 participants
- **Average cost to enter**.................. $3000 – $3500
- **Year it started**........................... 2007
- **Support offered**........................... Supported

The Yak Attack is one of the most challenging mountain bike races in the world, held annually in the rugged and remote regions of Nepal. Since its beginning in 2007, the race has attracted riders from around the globe. The event was founded to provide a unique racing experience that combines high-altitude cycling and the Nepalese way of life, traversing ancient trading routes and remote villages.

Spanning approximately 500km, the Yak Attack takes riders through some of the most demanding terrains on the planet. The course climbs to elevations of over 5416meters, including a pass through Thorong La, one of the world's highest navigable passes. The route covers a variety of challenging terrains from rocky trails and mud paths to snow-covered passes, making technical skills a necessity. The extreme altitude adds another layer of difficulty, with riders having to manage the risks of altitude sickness alongside physical exhaustion. The unpredictable weather of the Himalayas, ranging from intense sun to snow and biting cold, further challenges the participants, making this race a true test of endurance and resilience.

Entering the Yak Attack requires a blend of preparation and determination. Prospective racers should have experience in high-altitude mountain biking and be well-prepared for the physical challenges they will face. Registration is typically done online via the official Yak Attack website, where detailed information about race logistics, entry requirements, and fees are provided. Due to the extreme nature of the race and its remote location, entries are usually limited.

You can find more details about the Yak Attack on their official website:
https://www.mtb-worldwide.com/the-yak-attack/

ANDES PACIFICO

- **Location**.................................... Chile
- **Time of year**.............................. February
- **Approximate distance**................. 400km (249 miles)
- **Average time to finish**................ 5 days
- **Average number of entries**.......... 100 – 150 participants
- **Average cost to enter**.................. $1000 – $1500
- **Year it started**............................ 2014
- **Support offered**.......................... Supported

The Andes Pacifico is an exhilarating mountain bike enduro race that takes place annually in Chile. Launched in 2014, the event quickly gained popularity for offering one of the most challenging races in the world of mountain biking. Over the course of several days, participants traverse from the high Andes Mountains to the Pacific Ocean, experiencing a blend of breathtaking landscapes and diverse ecosystems that make the race not only a physical challenge but also a memorable one.

Spanning approximately five days, the race covers various terrains starting from the Andes mountains at altitudes over 3,500 meters and finishing at sea level by the Pacific Ocean. The course includes long descents with loose, rocky, and dry trails that challenge even the most skilled riders. Riders face a cumulative descent of tens of thousands of meters, testing their endurance and technical riding skills under extreme conditions. The dusty conditions, known as "anti-grip," make the bike handling extremely tricky. Each stage of the race offers something different, be that either the terrain and technical challenges.

Registration for the Andes Pacifico is open to both professional and amateur riders, with entries typically opening a few months before the event. Due to the demanding nature of the race, it is recommended that participants prepare adequately, ensuring they are well-versed in enduro racing and comfortable with the expected riding conditions.

You can find more details about the Andes Pacifico on their official website:
https://andespacificoenduro.com/

RUNNING

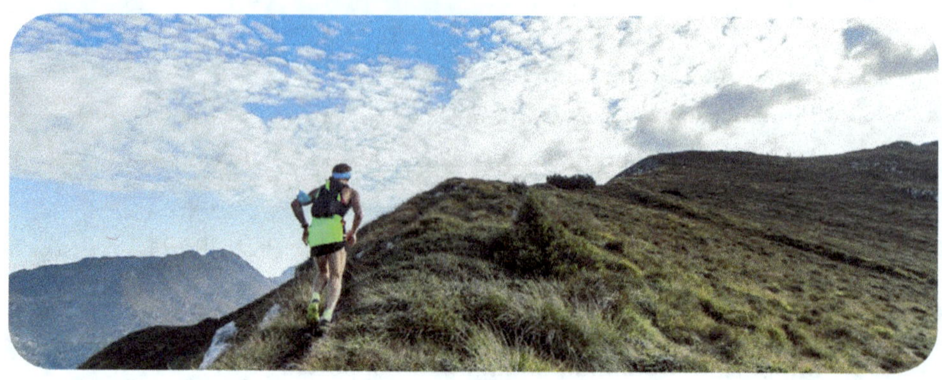

Running is a competitive sport where athletes race over various distances, aiming to complete a specified distance in the shortest possible time, with events typically categorized by distance or time. Due to the nature of ultra distance running events, the majority are trail races which occur on natural paths, adding elements of technical navigation and elevation changes. Each format challenges athletes' speed and endurance with the overarching goal of crossing the finish line ahead of their competitors.

The history of running as a competitive sport dates back to ancient civilizations. The earliest recorded races were part of the ancient Olympic Games in Greece, starting in 776 BC, where foot races were a central feature. The Greeks celebrated running as both a physical and cultural achievement, with events like the stadion (a short sprint) and the diaulos (a double-stadion race). During the Renaissance and early modern periods, running races began to be formalized in various countries, leading to the establishment of track and field events as we know them today. The 19th and 20th centuries saw the rise of modern athletics organizations, such as the International Association of Athletics Federations (IAAF), founded in 1912, which helped standardize rules and organize international competitions. Running has continued to evolve, with significant events such as the Boston Marathon, established in 1897, becoming iconic symbols of endurance and competition.

The concept of long endurance races in running began to take shape in the late 19th and early 20th centuries, as the sport of distance running became more organised and competitive. One of the earliest notable long-distance races is the marathon, inspired by the ancient Greek legend of Pheidippides, who is said to have run from the battlefield of Marathon to Athens to deliver news of victory. The modern marathon was introduced to the Olympic Games in 1896, with the first official race held in Athens.

Another early endurance race is the 24-hour race, which emerged in the early 20th century and challenged runners to cover the greatest distance possible within a 24-hour period. These events set the stage for the development of modern long-distance running and endurance racing, establishing benchmarks for distance and endurance in the sport.

Running races have become increasingly demanding as the sport has evolved, driven by advancements in training and race formats. Modern races often feature more challenging courses with varied terrain, including hills, trails, and extreme weather conditions. The rise of ultra-marathons, which cover distances beyond the traditional marathon, exemplifies this trend, with events like the Western States Endurance Run and the Ultra-Trail du Mont-Blanc pushing the limits of human endurance. Technological advancements, such as high-performance footwear have also enabled athletes to push their physical limits further, while the introduction of new race formats and challenges, such as obstacle course races and multi-day stage events, has added complexity to the sport. The increasing competitiveness of the field and the pursuit of new records of fastest known times (FKT) continue to drive the evolution of running races, making them even more challenging and varied.

When selecting what I believe to be the hardest running events in the world, I considered a variety of factors. While distance and elevation gain are obviously key, as with most endurance sports, running presents unique challenges. Being an impact-based sport with one of the highest injury rates, there's more to it than just covering long distances and steep climbs. Many of the races listed here feature diverse terrains, from mountain trails to snow-covered paths, which require significantly more energy than running on roads. These unstable surfaces also introduce the added risk of twisting an ankle or falling and getting injured, especially when fatigue sets in. With all these factors in mind, I've compiled a list of what I consider to be the world's toughest running races. Let's look at what's on offer.

SELF-TRANSCENDENCE RACE

- **Location**....................................... New York (United States)
- **Time of year**............................... July/ August
- **Approximate distance**................. 4989km (3100 miles)
- **Average time to finish**................ 40 – 52 days
- **Average number of entries**.......... 10 – 15 participants
- **Average cost to enter**................... Free
- **Year it started**............................. 1997
- **Support offered**........................... Supported

The Self-Transcendence 3100 mile Race, founded in 1997 by spiritual leader Sri Chinmoy, is known as the longest certified footrace in the world. This event is held annually in Queens, New York, and embodies the philosophy of self-transcendence, pushing the limits of what is possible physically and mentally. Sri Chinmoy believed that extreme physical challenges could offer spiritual benefits, helping participants to discover new possibilities within themselves. The race attracts ultra-endurance athletes who seek not only to test their physical limits but also to explore deeper spiritual and personal growth.

The course for the Self-Transcendence 3100 mile race is unusual by most ultramarathon standards. It consists of a single 0.5488 mile (883m) loop around a city block in Queens, New York. Runners must complete 5649 laps to reach the 3100-mile distance. The race takes place over 52 days, requiring participants to average at least 59.6 miles per day to finish within the time limit. The repetitive nature of the course, combined with the urban setting, summer heat, and the physical and mental fatigue of running nearly two marathons a day, makes this race uniquely challenging.

Entering the Self-Transcendence 3100 mile race requires a proven track record in multi-day ultramarathons, as the demands of the race are beyond those of typical endurance events. Potential entrants must demonstrate their ability to handle extreme distances over consecutive days. The selection process is careful to ensure that all participants are fully prepared for the physical and mental challenges of the race.

You can find info about the Self-transcendence race on their official website: https://3100.srichinmoyraces.org/

YUKON ARCTIC ULTRA

- **Location**..................................... Yukon (Canada)
- **Time of year**............................... February
- **Approximate distance**................. 640km (430 miles)
- **Average time to finish**................ 7 – 13 days
- **Average number of entries**.......... 50 participants
- **Average cost to enter**................... $2400
- **Year it started**............................ 2003
- **Support offered**........................... Semi-supported

The Yukon Arctic Ultra, often cited as the "world's coldest and toughest ultra," takes place annually in the Yukon Territory of Canada. The race started in 2003, branching off from the Yukon Quest, a famous dog sled race. It has since attracted a niche group of extreme athletes who seek to test their endurance against some of the harshest winter conditions on the planet. The race offers various distances, including marathon, 100-mile, 300-mile, and even a 430-mile version, each presenting unique challenges and requiring significant mental and physical preparation.

The Yukon Arctic Ultra follows the Yukon Quest trail, one of the most remote and unforgiving environments in the North American wilderness. Depending on the distance, competitors may travel from Whitehorse to checkpoints like Braeburn, Carmacks, Pelly Crossing, and Dawson City. Participants face extreme cold, with temperatures often dropping below -30°C, and sometimes as low as -40°C or colder, combined with potential winds and snowfall. The trail conditions can vary dramatically from packed snow to icy patches, which can be treacherous underfoot. The remoteness of the route means that participants must be self-sufficient, capable of handling extreme cold, and prepared to survive potentially life-threatening conditions.

Entering the Yukon Arctic Ultra requires thorough preparation in terms of physical conditioning, cold-weather survival skills, and appropriate gear. Potential participants should have experience in cold-weather endurance events and must submit a detailed application showcasing their qualifications and readiness for the race.

You can find more details about the Yukon Arctic Ultra on their official website:
https://arcticultra.de/

THE SPINE RACE

- **Location**... United Kingdom
- **Time of year**................................. January
- **Approximate distance**.................. 430km (268 miles)
- **Average time to finish**................. 7 – 14 days
- **Average number of entries**.......... 150 – 200 participants
- **Average cost to enter**................... $500 – $600
- **Year it started**............................. 2012
- **Support offered**........................... Supported

The Spine Race is a renowned ultra-endurance race known for its extreme challenge and terrain. First held in 2012, the race was inspired by the desire to push the limits of endurance running in the UK's wildest landscapes. Officially named the Montane Spine Race due to sponsorship, it traverses the Pennine Way, one of the UK's most iconic long-distance trails. The event quickly gained a reputation for its demanding nature, attracting elite and amateur endurance athletes from around the world. The race is celebrated for its brutal physical and mental demands.

The Spine Race follows the Pennine Way from its southern start in Edale, Derbyshire, to its northern terminus in Kirk Yetholm, Scottish Borders. The trail is renowned for its terrain, which includes steep ascents and descents, rocky paths, and boggy moorland. What sets the Spine Race apart is its winter timing, which subjects participants to severe weather conditions including freezing temperatures, snow, ice, and rain. This creates a treacherous environment where visibility and traction can be severely compromised, significantly increasing the difficulty of the race. The course also features considerable elevation gain, with runners navigating the Pennine Hills and the Cheviot Hills, while being self-sufficient, carrying all necessary equipment and supplies.

Entering the Spine Race involves meeting stringent entry criteria designed to ensure that participants are well-prepared for the event's extreme demands. Applicants must have a proven track record in ultra-endurance running or similar challenging events, often requiring previous completion of races of at least 100 miles or similar endurance feats.

You can find more details about the Spine Race on their official website: https://www.thespinerace.com/

MOAB 240

- **Location**..................................... Utah (United States)
- **Time of year**............................. October
- **Approximate distance**................. 386km (240 miles)
- **Average time to finish**................. 80 – 112 hours
- **Average number of entries**........... 150 – 200 participants
- **Average cost to enter**................... $1200 – $1400
- **Year it started**............................. 2015
- **Support offered**........................... Supported

The Moab 240 is an ultra-endurance race renowned for its extreme length and challenging conditions. The event covers a staggering distance of approximately 240 miles across some of the most visually spectacular terrain in the American Southwest. It was designed to push the limits of human endurance, combining high elevation, challenging trails, and variable weather conditions. The race has become a benchmark for ultra-endurance athletes, drawing competitors from around the world who seek to test their limits.

The route includes significant elevation changes, with runners ascending and descending over 28,000 feet (8500 meters) throughout the race. The terrain varies from technical single-track trails to rocky paths and sandy stretches. The high elevation areas can lead to altitude-related challenges, and the remote nature of the course means that support is limited, and self-sufficiency is crucial. The race typically spans multiple days and nights, demanding not only physical stamina but also mental resilience and strategic pacing. Weather conditions in Moab can be extreme, ranging from scorching daytime temperatures to cold nights. This combination of distance, elevation gain, technical terrain, and harsh environmental conditions makes the Moab 240 one of the most gruelling ultra-endurance races in the world.

To enter the Moab 240, participants are generally required to have a proven track record in ultra-endurance events, including previous completions of races of at least 100 miles or more. Participants must also adhere to specific gear and equipment standards, including cold-weather clothing, navigation tools, and survival gear, as the race traverses remote and rugged areas.

You can find more details about the Moab 240 on their official website: https://www.destinationtrailrun.com/moab

TOR DES GÉANTS

- **Location**...................................... Italy
- **Time of year**............................... September
- **Approximate distance**................. 330km (205 miles)
- **Average time to finish**................ 70 – 100 hours
- **Average number of entries**.......... 1100 participants
- **Average cost to enter**.................. $700
- **Year it started**............................ 2010
- **Support offered**........................... Semi-supported

The Tor des Géants, known as the Tour of Giants, is one of the most prestigious endurance races that takes place annually in the heart of the Italian Alps, within the Aosta Valley. Since 2010, the event has captivated ultra-endurance athletes from around the globe with its breathtaking scenery. This non-stop race encompasses the entire region around the Alps, weaving through the Gran Paradiso National Park and Mont Avic Regional Park. The race is designed not only as a physical challenge but also as an exploration of the region, providing runners with an immersive experience in the mountainous landscapes.

The Tor des Géants covers an impressive 330km (205 miles) with a staggering 78,740ft (24,000 meters) of cumulative elevation gain. The route traverses mountainous terrain, featuring high altitude passes, challenging climbs, and technical descents. Participants encounter varied conditions including potentially extreme weather from intense sun to chilling temperatures, adding to the race's difficulty.

Entry into the Tor des Géants is highly competitive, involving a selection process that often includes a lottery due to the high demand and limited spots. Prospective participants must register their interest and comply with specific qualifications to ensure they can endure such an extreme event. The race typically fills quickly, with runners from all corners of the globe eager to take on the challenge.

You can find more details about the Tor des Géants on their official website:
https://www.torxtrail.com/tor-des-géants®

GRAND TO GRAND ULTRA

- **Location**... United States
- **Time of year**................................. September
- **Approximate distance**.................. 273km (170 miles)
- **Average time to finish**................. 6 – 7 days
- **Average number of entries**.......... 100 – 150 participants
- **Average cost to enter**................... $3400
- **Year it started**.............................. 2012
- **Support offered**............................ Unsupported

The Grand to Grand Ultra is a self-supported stage race that takes runners on a journey from the North Rim of the Grand Canyon to the Grand Staircase in Utah. Launched in 2012, it has quickly become renowned as one of the most demanding and scenic ultramarathon events in the world. The race is unique not only because of its stunning landscapes but also due to its format, which emphasizes self-sufficiency and endurance over varying terrain.

Covering approximately 170 miles (273km) over six stages, the Grand to Grand Ultra is recognized for its formidable course that ascends from the depths of the Grand Canyon to the heights of the Grand Staircase. The route crosses many diverse landscapes, including desert sands, rocky trails, and steep dunes, culminating in a total elevation gain of over 18,000ft. The variability of the terrain, combined with the challenges of self-sufficiency where runners must carry their own gear, food, and sleeping equipment adds to the difficulty. The desert climate also plays a significant role, with daytime temperatures soaring and nights that can be surprisingly cold, testing the runners' ability to endure.

Prospective participants looking to enter need to demonstrate endurance experience or a strong athletic background due to the rigorous demands of the race. Registration is typically done through the official website, where detailed information about the necessary qualifications, race rules, and equipment requirements can be found.

You can find more info about the Grand to Grand Ultra on their official website: https://g2gultra.com/

MARATHON DES SABLES

- **Location**.. Morocco
- **Time of year**............................... April
- **Approximate distance**................. 250km (155 miles)
- **Average time to finish**................ 20 – 50 hours
- **Average number of entries**.......... 1000 participants
- **Average cost to enter**.................. $2500 – $3500
- **Year it started**............................. 1986
- **Support offered**........................... Semi-supported

The Marathon des Sables, often referred to simply as MdS, is a legendary ultra-marathon that is considered one of the toughest foot races on Earth. First held in 1986, the event was created by French concert promoter Patrick Bauer, who was inspired by his solo traverse of the Sahara Desert two years earlier. The race has since grown in notoriety, attracting thousands of runners from around the world who come to test their limits in one of the most inhospitable climates on the planet. The MdS spans over six days and covers approximately 250km through the Moroccan Sahara, challenging participants with extreme heat, arduous terrain, and the daunting task of self-sufficiency.

The course takes runners across a wide variety of desert landscapes including rocky plains, rugged mountains, sand dunes, and dry riverbeds, each presenting its own set of challenges. Temperatures can soar to over 50degrees Celsius during the day and plummeting to near freezing at night. Competitors must carry all their own equipment and supplies for the duration of the race, including food, sleeping gear, and medical supplies, with the only assistance from race organizers being the provision of water and a tent for overnight shelter.

Entering requires careful planning and preparation, as spots in the race are highly sought after and often sell out quickly. Prospective participants must register well in advance and are usually subjected to a selection process that includes an assessment of their readiness for such an extreme event. The race also has a substantial entry fee, which includes medical support, water supply and communal Berber tents for sleeping.

You can find more info about the Marathon Des Sables on their official website: http://www.marathondessables.com

SPARTATHLON

- **Location**.. Greece
- **Time of year**................................ September
- **Approximate distance**................. 250km (155 miles)
- **Average time to finish**................ 20 – 36 hours
- **Average number of entries**.......... 390 participants
- **Average cost to enter**................... $550
- **Year it started**............................. 1982
- **Support offered**........................... Supported

The Spartathlon is one of the most historic and challenging ultra-marathon races in the world, tracing the footsteps of Pheidippides, an ancient Athenian long-distance runner who, according to legend, was sent to Sparta in 490 BC to seek help against the Persians in the Battle of Marathon. The race was conceived in 1982, following British RAF Wing Commander John Foden and two fellow officers' successful attempt to test the feasibility of covering the distance in a single day. The following year, the official Spartathlon was born, quickly becoming a cornerstone event in the ultrarunning community, revered not only for its gruelling challenge but also for its deep historical roots.

Spanning approximately 246km (153 miles) from Athens to Sparta, the course of the Spartathlon is notorious for its difficulty. It begins at the Acropolis, winding through the streets of Athens, before heading into the more isolated terrains of the Peloponnesian countryside. Runners face a formidable climb over the mountainous Sangas Pass at night, contending with steep ascents and potentially hazardous weather conditions. The race continues through ancient vineyards and olive groves, demanding speed and endurance to beat the 36-hour cut-off time, all under the Mediterranean sun.

Entry into the Spartathlon is highly competitive, requiring athletes to meet stringent qualifying standards based on performance in other ultramarathons. Prospective participants must apply through the race's official website, where they can also find detailed information on qualifying criteria, race rules, and preparation tips. Registration typically opens in the spring, and due to the popularity and prestige of the race, securing a spot can be as challenging as the event itself.

You can find more details about the Spartathlon race on their official website:
https://www.spartathlon.gr/en/home/

JUNGLE ULTRA

- **Location**.. Peru (Amazon rainforest)
- **Time of year**............................... June
- **Approximate distance**................. 230km (143 miles)
- **Average time to finish**................ 5 – 7 days
- **Average number of entries**.......... 40 – 80 participants
- **Average cost to enter**.................. $3500 – $4000
- **Year it started**............................ 2011
- **Support offered**........................... Unsupported

The Jungle Ultra is an exhilarating and extreme endurance race that puts participants deep into the Peruvian Amazon Rainforest. This event is designed to push the limits of human endurance through one of the most biodiverse environments on the planet. Participants experience the jungle, with dense forests to fast-flowing rivers, all while navigating a course that tests everything including their survival skills. The race, which has been attracting runners for many years, aims to provide a unique experience that goes beyond conventional marathons or trail runs.

Covering approximately 230km, the Jungle Ultra course is marked by a series of complex challenges. The terrain includes muddy jungle trails, river crossings, and steep, slippery ascents. Competitors must contend with high humidity and temperatures that can soar to over 30°C (86°F) during the day, dropping to near freezing at night. The race is also self-supported, meaning runners must carry all their own supplies, including food and safety equipment, while managing their hydration with water provided only at checkpoints. The combination of harsh environmental conditions, self-sufficiency requirements, and the mental strain of isolation in the jungle makes this race particularly arduous.

Participants are typically required to demonstrate experience in ultra-distance running before they can enter, and they must be prepared for the self-sufficient aspects of the race. Registration details, race rules, and preparation guidelines can be found on the official Beyond the Ultimate website, which organizes the Jungle Ultra among other extreme races.

You can find more information about the Jungle Ultra on their official website:
https://www.beyondtheultimate.co.uk/race/jungle-ultra/

BADWATER 135

- **Location**.................................... California (United States)
- **Time of year**.............................. July
- **Approximate distance**................. 217km (135 miles)
- **Average time to finish**................. 24 – 48 hours
- **Average number of entries**.......... 100 participants
- **Average cost to enter**................... $1500
- **Year it started**............................. 1987
- **Support offered**........................... Supported

The Badwater 135 is known as one of the most extreme running races in the world, known specifically for its gruelling distance and harsh environmental conditions. It officially started in 1987, and the race takes place annually in Death Valley, California, one of the hottest places on Earth. It is named after Badwater Basin, the lowest point in North America, which marks the starting point of the race. Over the years, Badwater 135 has attracted ultra-marathoners from across the globe seeking to test their limits in a race that has become synonymous with extreme endurance.

Spanning 135 miles, the course runs from Badwater Basin in Death Valley at 282ft (86 meters) below sea level to Whitney Portal at the base of Mount Whitney, at an elevation of 8360ft (2548 meters). The race takes place in mid-July, when temperatures can soar up to 130 degrees Fahrenheit (54 degrees Celsius), challenging runners with not only the heat but also the rough, arid terrain of the desert. The course encompasses three mountain ranges, totalling 14,600 feet (4450 meters) of cumulative vertical ascent and 6,100 feet (1859 meters) of cumulative descent, which is a lot even for the most seasoned ultra-runners.

Entry into the Badwater 135 is highly competitive, with participants typically required to have completed at least three qualifying events and demonstrate experience in handling extreme conditions. The race also mandates a comprehensive application that includes an essay and a resume of ultra-running experience.

You can find more information about the Badwater135 on their official website:
http://www.badwater.com/event/badwater-135/

ULTRA TRAIL DU MONT BLANC

- **Location**.. Europe (France, Italy & Switzerland)
- **Time of year**............................... August
- **Approximate distance**................. 171km (106 miles)
- **Average time to finish**................ 20 – 46 hours
- **Average number of entries**.......... 2300 participants
- **Average cost to enter**................... $200 – $300
- **Year it started**............................. 2003
- **Support offered**........................... Supported

The Ultra-Trail du Mont-Blanc (UTMB) is one of the most prestigious ultra-marathon events globally, held annually in the Alps. Originating in 2003, the race has grown significantly, drawing thousands of runners to it's start line. The event was born from the passion of its founders, Michel and Catherine Poletti, who envisioned a race that encapsulated the spirit of mountain and trail running across international borders.

UTMB's course is notorious for its difficulty, covering approximately 171km with a staggering 10,000 meters of cumulative elevation gain. The route encircles Mont Blanc, passing through three countries and incorporating high altitudes, varied terrains, and often unpredictable weather conditions. These elements combine to test even the most seasoned ultra-runners, making it a coveted title in the trail running community.

Entry into UTMB is highly competitive, requiring runners to accumulate points from other qualifying races and then participate in a lottery system due to the high demand.

You can find more information about the UTMB on their official website:
https://montblanc.utmb.world/races/UTMB

HARDROCK HUNDRED

- **Location**.. Colorado (United States)
- **Time of year**.................................. July
- **Approximate distance**.................. 161km (100 miles)
- **Average time to finish**................ 30 – 48 hours
- **Average number of entries**.......... 145 participants
- **Average cost to enter**................... $325
- **Year it started**............................. 1992
- **Support offered**........................... Supported

The Hardrock Hundred Mile Endurance Run, established in 1992, is more than just an ultramarathon; it's a test of resilience against the rugged backdrop of Colorado's San Juan Mountains. Originally designed to link the region's historic mining towns, Hardrock celebrates the legacy and adventure of the 1800s mining era through a course that mirrors the arduous journeys miners endured back then.

The Hardrock Hundred features a 100-mile loop with 33,000ft of cumulative elevation gain and an equal amount of descent, capped with a 48hr cut off time. The course navigates steep climbs, technical trails, and high altitudes above 12,000ft, including a crossing at Handies Peak at over 14,000ft. The terrain and unpredictable mountain weather add layers of complexity, making it one of the most demanding ultramarathons globally.

Entry into the Hardrock Hundred is highly competitive, managed through a lottery system due to its limited slots. Aspiring participants must meet specific qualifying criteria, reflecting experience with similar trail races.

You can find more details about the Hardrock Hundred on their official website:
https://hardrock100.com/

BARKLEY MARATHON

- **Location**.. Tennessee (United States)
- **Time of year**................................. March/ April
- **Approximate distance**................. 160km (100 miles)
- **Average time to finish**................. 60 hours
- **Average number of entries**.......... 40 participants
- **Average cost to enter**................... $1.50
- **Year it started**.............................. 1986
- **Support offered**............................ Unsupported

The Barkley Marathons is an ultra-marathon trail race held annually in Frozen Head State Park, Tennessee, and is known for being one of the most challenging endurance races in the world. Created in 1986 by Gary "Lazarus Lake" Cantrell, the event was inspired by a 1977 prison escape from the nearby Brushy Mountain State Penitentiary. The escapee covered only 8 miles in 55 hours, which prompted Cantrell to design a race that he believed could test the limits of human endurance over a 100mile course. The Barkley is notorious not only for its physical difficulty but also for its secretive and unconventional application process that adds to its mystique.

The course consists of a 20mile unmarked loop (though participants argue it is longer), which must be completed five times for a total of 100 miles. The race features no aid stations and requires runners to navigate through thick brush, steep climbs, and deadly descents, accumulating over 60,000ft of elevation gain throughout the race. The course is also known for its harsh weather conditions, ranging from freezing temperatures to sweltering humidity. Each loop includes navigating to find hidden books from which runners must tear a page corresponding to their bib number to prove they completed the route. This unique element, combined with physical and navigational challenges, ensures that most years see few, if any, finishers.

Entry into the Barkley Marathons is as enigmatic as the race itself. Hopeful participants must complete an application process shrouded in secrecy, with requirements and deadlines that are not publicly disclosed. Applicants need to submit an essay on why they should be allowed to race, and entry fees are famously low, supplemented by a license plate from the applicant's state or country, or whatever odd item the race director requests that year. The application process is intentionally opaque, part of what adds to the allure and challenge of the Barkley. There is no official website maintained by the race.

WESTERN STATES ENDURANCE RUN

- **Location**....................................... California (United States)
- **Time of year**............................... June
- **Approximate distance**................. 160km (100 miles)
- **Average time to finish**................ 24 – 30 hours
- **Average number of entries**.......... 370 participants
- **Average cost to enter**.................... $410
- **Year it started**............................. 1974
- **Support offered**........................... Supported

The Western States Endurance Run, established in 1974, has the distinction of being the world's oldest 100-mile trail race. Originating from a horse race along the Western States Trail, it transformed into an endurance run after Gordy Ainsleigh joined the horses in 1974 to complete the course on foot, proving the potential for a foot race along the same rugged terrain.

Spanning from Squaw Valley to Auburn, California, the Western States course covers 100 miles of challenging trails through the Sierra Nevada Mountains. It features a cumulative ascent of over 18,000ft and a descent of 23,000ft, confronting runners with extreme temperatures, technical terrain, and high altitudes, making it one of the most gruelling endurance challenges in the sport.

Entry into the Western States Endurance Run is primarily through a lottery system due to its popularity and limited race spots. Runners must qualify by completing an approved 100-mile race within the stipulated times to be eligible for the lottery.

You can find more information about the Western States endurance run on their official website: https://www.wser.org/

TRIATHLON

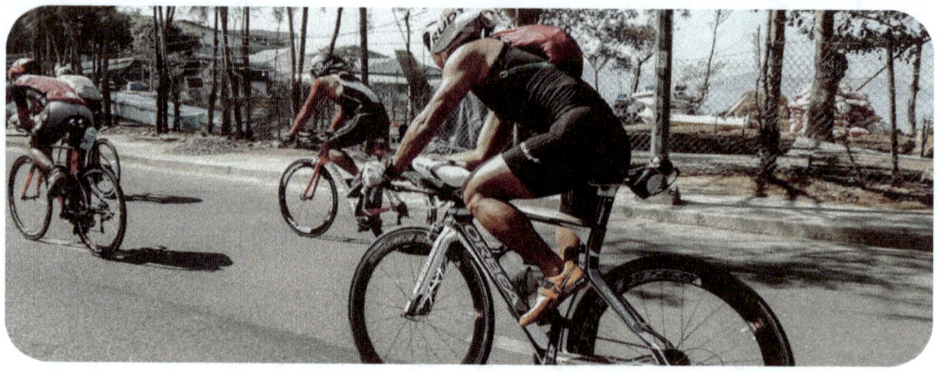

Triathlon racing is a multi-discipline endurance sport that combines swimming, cycling, and running in a single event, with competitors transitioning between each segment to complete the race. Races are typically structured with a swim segment followed by a bike ride and concluding with a run, all performed consecutively without breaks. The sport features various distances, from sprint triathlons, which are shorter and more accessible, to Ironman and half-Ironman races, which require extensive training.

Triathlon as a structured sport originated in the early 1970s, building on the concept of combining different endurance disciplines. The first organized triathlon race took place in 1974 in San Diego, California, known as the "Mission Bay Triathlon," which featured a 400-meter swim, a 8km bike, and a 5km run. This event marked the beginning of triathlon as a competitive sport, though the concept of multi-sport challenges existed in various forms throughout history. The sport gained popularity rapidly, and in 1982, the first Ironman race was held in Hawaii, featuring a 3.8km swim, a 180km bike ride, and a 42km marathon run. This race set a standard for long-distance triathlon and established the Ironman brand. Over the following decades, triathlon evolved with the establishment of governing bodies like the International Triathlon Union (ITU) and the inclusion of the sport in the Olympic Games in 2000, further cementing its place in the global athletic community.

Triathlon races have become increasingly challenging due to advancements in equipment, evolving race formats, and the growing competitiveness of the sport. Modern races often feature more demanding courses with varied terrain, including mountainous bike routes and technical running trails. The introduction of extreme distance events, such as the Ultraman, which extends beyond traditional Ironman distances, increases the difficulty of what events are out there.

Technological advancements in gear, such as aerodynamic bikes, advanced wetsuits, and high-performance running shoes, have pushed athletes to achieve higher speeds and tackle more challenging conditions. Additionally, the rise of multi-sport events and varied race formats, including triathlons with unique combinations of swim, bike, and run segments or multi-day challenges, has added an excitement to the sport.

The difficulty of a triathlon race is shaped by a combination of factors. Physically, athletes must manage the demands of three distinct disciplines which each requiring different energy systems and muscle groups. The transitions between these disciplines also present challenges, as athletes must quickly switch from one activity to another while maintaining speed. Psychologically, the race requires mental toughness to overcome fatigue, maintain focus, and strategically pace oneself throughout the event. The combination of these elements makes triathlon racing a rigorous test of endurance and skill.

Triathlons are particularly hard to categorize when determining the most difficult events. Once the distance exceeds the Ironman, race formats become highly variable. Some events take place over multiple days, with each discipline on separate days, while others rearrange the typical swim, bike, and run order. Environmental factors greatly influence the difficulty as well, with the freezing temperatures of the Norseman or the Enduroman's English Channel swim being particularly notable. The races in this chapter are some of the most extreme and undoubtedly rank among the toughest triathlons in the world. Enjoy!

THE EPIC5 CLASSIC

- **Location**.. Hawaii (United States)
- **Time of year**................................... May
- **Approximate distance**................. 5 Ironman's in 5 days
- **Average time to finish**................. 12 – 16 hours (per day)
- **Average number of entries**.......... 12 participants
- **Average cost to enter**................... $5000 – $7000
- **Year it started**............................. 2010
- **Support offered**........................... Supported

The EPIC5 Challenge was designed by Jason Lester and Rich Roll in 2010 as an ultimate endurance test, designed to push the limits of even the most seasoned triathletes. The desire was to create an extreme physical and mental challenge that also showcases the beauty of the Hawaiian Islands. EPIC5 has since, gained a reputation as one of the most demanding multi-day endurance events in the world, attracting athletes who are looking to test their limits in some of the most beautiful places on earth.

The course involves completing five full Ironman-distance triathlons on five different Hawaiian Islands over five consecutive days. The race begins on Kauai and moves through Oahu, Molokai, Maui, and concludes on the Big Island. The logistical challenge of moving between islands nightly adds a layer of complexity when coupled with the varied climates and terrains of each island, from the rugged coastlines to volcanic mountains.

Entry into the EPIC5 Challenge requires a proven track record of completion in long-distance triathlons, specifically Ironman or similar events. Potential participants must submit a detailed application showcasing their endurance race history, physical fitness, and mental preparedness. Due to the extreme nature of the race and the limited slots available, a comprehensive review of each application is conducted to ensure that all participants are capable of safely completing the challenge. Prospective athletes are encouraged to have a strong support system and the ability to commit to rigorous training in preparation for the event.

You can find more details about the Epic5 Classic on their official website:
https://www.epic5.com/epic5-classic

BRETZEL ULTRA QUINTUPLE TRIATHLON

- **Location**.. France
- **Time of year**.................................... July
- **Approximate distance**.................. 19km swim, 900km bike,
  211km run12
- **Average time to finish**.................. 148 hours
- **Average number of entries**.......... 30 – 50 participants
- **Average cost to enter**................... $1200 – $1500
- **Year it started**.............................. N/A
- **Support offered**........................... Supported

The Bretzel Ultra Quintuple Triathlon is an extreme endurance event set in the scenic Alsace region of France. This event pushes the boundaries of endurance racing with a race format that multiplies the classic Ironman distances by five. Designed for the most seasoned athletes, this race offers an extraordinary challenge that tests stamina and mental strength. It attracts a select group of ultra-endurance athletes every year from around the world who are drawn to its unique demands.

The course of the Bretzel Ultra Quintuple Triathlon is designed to be as gruelling as it is picturesque. The race begins with a 19km swim in Lac de Kruth, followed by a 900km bike segment that winds through the demanding terrain of the Vosges Mountains, incorporating significant elevation changes that challenge even the most seasoned of cyclists. The race concludes with a 211km run through the rolling hills and vineyards of Alsace, providing a stunning backdrop to the exhausting final leg. The repetitive nature of the laps, combined with the physical toll of continuous long-distance efforts over several days, adds a profound level of difficulty to the race.

Entry into the Bretzel Ultra Quintuple Triathlon is highly selective, requiring athletes to demonstrate exceptional endurance capabilities and experience in similar ultra-endurance events. Potential participants must provide a detailed sports resume, including results from previous ultra-distance races or other significant endurance achievements. The organizers scrutinize these qualifications to ensure that all entrants possess the necessary physical conditioning to safely compete in this extreme event.

You can find details about the Bretzel Ultra Triathlon on their official website:
https://bretzelultratri.com/en/quintuple-continuous-day/

ENDUROMAN

- **Location**.. United Kingdom & France
- **Time of year**............................... June – September
- **Approximate distance**................. 140km run, 33km swim, 291km bike
- **Average time to finish**................. 60 – 90 hours
- **Average number of entries**.......... 30 participants
- **Average cost to enter**................... $3000 – $4000
- **Year it started**.............................. 2001
- **Support offered**........................... Supported

The Enduroman Arch to Arc is an ultra-triathlon that stands out as one of the most arduous endurance challenges in the world. It was created in 2001 to push the boundaries of human endurance racing. The race uniquely combines running, swimming, and cycling across two of Europe's most iconic cities. It not only tests physical endurance but also logistical planning.

The course of the Enduroman Arch to Arc is notorious for its extreme demands. Starting with a 140km run from London's Marble Arch to the coast in Dover, athletes then face one of the most challenging parts of the race, swimming 33km across the notoriously unpredictable English Channel. Once in France, the race concludes with a 291km bike ride from Calais to the Arc de Triomphe in Paris. The difficulty is compounded by the logistics of timing the swim with favourable tides and weather, alongside the physical challenge of transitioning between disciplines without significant rest.

Entry into the Enduroman Arch to Arc is selective and requires proof of capability to handle such a demanding multi-sport event. Interested athletes must submit an application detailing their experience and qualifications in ultra-endurance sports. The race directors review these applications to ensure that all participants are suitably prepared for the physical and mental challenges they will face.

You can find more information about the Enduroman on their official website: https://enduroman.com/

THE ULTRAMAN CANADA

- **Location**..................................... Canada
- **Time of year**.............................. July
- **Approximate distance**................. 10km swim, 421.1km bike,
  84.3km run
- **Average time to finish**................. 3 days
- **Average number of entries**.......... 40 participants
- **Average cost to enter**................... $1800 – $2000
- **Year it started**............................ 1993
- **Support offered**.......................... Supported

Ultraman Canada, first held in 1993 in Penticton, like many others in this book is part of the global Ultraman series, a collection of ultra-endurance triathlon events that push the limits of endurance racing. Originally founded to create an event that was more personal and challenging than the conventional Ironman, Ultraman Canada established itself as a premier race in the Ultraman community. It is celebrated for its breathtaking scenery, community support, and the spirit it fosters among participants and volunteers alike.

The course of Ultraman Canada is renowned for its stunning yet challenging terrain. Day 1 starts with a 10km swim in the clear, fresh waters of Okanagan Lake, followed by a 145.1km bike ride through rolling hills. Day 2 tests cyclists with a gruelling 276km bike route that showcases the landscapes of British Columbia. The final day features an 84.3km double marathon run along the scenic routes surrounding Penticton. The race's difficulty is compounded by the cumulative fatigue athletes face across three days of extreme endurance racing, combined with potential variable weather conditions, including high heat or rain.

To enter Ultraman Canada, athletes must demonstrate significant experience in endurance events, specifically in completing at least one Ironman-distance event or a comparable long-course triathlon. Applicants are required to submit a detailed sports resume along with their registration. Acceptance into the race is selective to ensure that all competitors can safely meet the demands of the three-day endurance challenge.

You can find more details about the Ultraman Canada on their official website: https://officialultramancanada.com/

THE ULTRAMAN AUSTRALIA

- **Location**..................................... Australia
- **Time of year**............................... May
- **Approximate distance**................. 10km swim, 421.1km bike, 84.3km run
- **Average time to finish**................ 3 days
- **Average number of entries**.......... 50 participants
- **Average cost to enter**.................. $1800 – $2000
- **Year it started**............................ 2015
- **Support offered**.......................... Supported

Ultraman Canada, first held in 1993 in Penticton, like many others in this book is part of the global Ultraman series, a collection of ultra-endurance triathlon events that push the limits of endurance racing. Originally founded to create an event that was more personal and challenging than the conventional Ironman, Ultraman Canada established itself as a premier race in the Ultraman community. It is celebrated for its breathtaking scenery, community support, and the spirit it fosters among participants and volunteers alike.

The course of Ultraman Canada is renowned for its stunning yet challenging terrain. Day 1 starts with a 10km swim in the clear, fresh waters of Okanagan Lake, followed by a 145.1km bike ride through rolling hills. Day 2 tests cyclists with a gruelling 276km bike route that showcases the landscapes of British Columbia. The final day features an 84.3km double marathon run along the scenic routes surrounding Penticton. The race's difficulty is compounded by the cumulative fatigue athletes face across three days of extreme endurance racing, combined with potential variable weather conditions, including high heat or rain.

To enter Ultraman Canada, athletes must demonstrate significant experience in endurance events, specifically in completing at least one Ironman-distance event or a comparable long-course triathlon. Applicants are required to submit a detailed sports resume along with their registration. Acceptance into the race is selective to ensure that all competitors can safely meet the demands of the three-day endurance challenge.

You can find more details about the Ultraman Canada on their official website:
https://officialultramancanada.com/

AUSTRIA EXTREME TRIATHLON

- **Location**...................................... Austria
- **Time of year**.............................. June
- **Approximate distance**................. 3.8km swim, 186km bike, 44km run
- **Average time to finish**................. 12 – 17 hours
- **Average number of entries**.......... 300 participants
- **Average cost to enter**................... $500 – $700
- **Year it started**............................. 2015
- **Support offered**........................... Supported

The Austria Extreme Triathlon is a celebrated event in the world of extreme sports. Launched in 2015, this race quickly gained a reputation as one of the toughest yet most rewarding triathlons in Europe. It attracts athletes who are not only looking to test their physical limits but also to experience one of the most picturesque landscapes Austria has to offer.

The Austria Extreme Triathlon's course is renowned for its formidable difficulty. The race begins with a 3.8km swim in the chilly waters of the Kopfstausee, followed by a 186km bike ride that features over 3800 meters of elevation gain through the Styrian mountains. The final leg is a 44km run, which includes a steep ascent to the iconic Dachstein mountain. The combination of distance, elevation gain, and potential for variable alpine weather conditions makes this race a supreme test of endurance and willpower.

To enter the Austria Extreme Triathlon, athletes must demonstrate experience in long-distance triathlons or similar endurance events. The registration process typically involves an application where athletes provide details about their previous race history and preparedness for the extreme demands of the course. Due to the challenging nature of the race, it is recommended that participants have substantial experience in handling tough terrain and harsh weather conditions. This ensures that all entrants are fully capable of completing the race safely and within the required time limits.

You can find info about the Austria Extreme Triathlon on their official website: https://www.autxtri.com/en

NORSEMAN

- **Location**.. Norway
- **Time of year**.............................. August
- **Approximate distance**................. 3.8km swim, 180km bike, 42.2km run
- **Average time to finish**................. 11 – 16 hours
- **Average number of entries**.......... 250 – 300 participants
- **Average cost to enter**................... $750
- **Year it started**............................. 2003
- **Support offered**........................... Semi-supported

The Norseman Xtreme Triathlon is renowned as one of the most challenging and unique long-distance triathlons in the world. Established in 2003, it was designed to be a test of endurance and resilience in the raw environment of Norway. The race starts with a jump from a ferry into cold and dark waters of Eidfjord and challenges athletes to push their limits across some of the most demanding terrain in Scandinavia.

The Norseman course begins with a 3.8km swim in the waters of Hardangerfjord, followed by a 180km bike ride that includes several mountain passes, and concludes with a full marathon ending at the rocky summit of Gaustatoppen, one of Norway's highest peaks. The total elevation gain during the race is substantial, with the run segment alone featuring a climb of over 1800 meters. The unpredictable weather, ranging from roasting sun to chilling winds and rain, adds to the race's difficulty. This gruelling combination of distance, elevation, and weather makes Norseman a supreme test of endurance.

Entry into the Norseman Xtreme Triathlon is highly competitive, with selection via a lottery system due to the limited slots and high demand. Hopeful participants must apply within the designated entry period and can choose to enter either individually or as part of a team. Those not selected in the lottery have a chance to win a slot through various contests and charity auctions held by the organizers.

You can find more info about the Norseman triathlon on their official website: https://nxtri.com/

SWISSMAN

- **Location**.............................. Switzerland
- **Time of year**............................... June
- **Approximate distance**.................. 3.8km swim, 180km bike, 42.2km run
- **Average time to finish**.................. 12 – 15 hours
- **Average number of entries**.......... 250 participants
- **Average cost to enter**................... $550 – $750
- **Year it started**............................. 2013
- **Support offered**........................... Supported

The Swissman Xtreme Triathlon is a point-to-point adventure triathlon that takes athletes on a journey across some of the most iconic landscapes in Switzerland. Started in 2013, Swissman is part of the XTRI World Tour, a series of extreme triathlons around the globe. Unlike traditional triathlons, Swissman offers a unique experience with limited participant numbers to preserve the personal challenge.

Swissman begins with a swim in Lake Maggiore, followed by a bike ride through the Swiss Alps, featuring several mountain passes, and concludes with a marathon that ends at the base of the Eiger North Face. The race has over 3500 meters of altitude gain on the bike and an additional 1800 meters during the run. The demanding elevation, coupled with potentially variable weather conditions, make Swissman a formidable challenge for even the most seasoned triathletes.

Entry into the Swissman Xtreme Triathlon is conducted through a lottery system due to its limited spots and high demand. Athletes interested in participating need to register for the lottery within the designated period. Comprehensive details about the entry process, race conditions, and preparation tips are available on the official Swissman website.

You can find more info about the Swissman triathlon on their official website:
https://suixtri.com/en/

OBSTACLE COURSE RACING

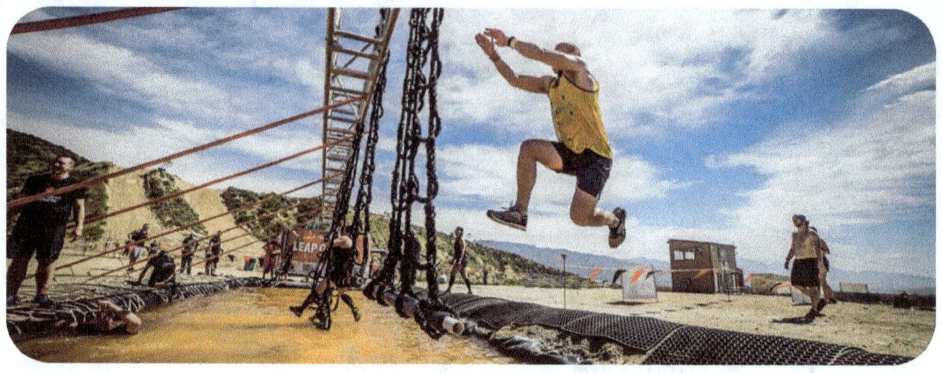

Obstacle course racing (OCR) is a sport that combines running with a series of physical challenges or obstacles set along a course. These races typically involve a mix of terrain, including mud, water and obstacles such as climbing walls, rope swings, monkey bars, and crawls. Competitors are required to complete each obstacle, and failing to do so often results in penalties, such as additional physical tasks or time penalties. OCR events vary in distance and difficulty, from short sprints to lengthy endurance races that can exceed 20 miles. The races are designed to test a wide range of skills, including strength, agility, endurance, and problem-solving. The integration of obstacles into running courses not only challenges physical capabilities but also demands strategic planning and adaptability as participants move through often unpredictable conditions.

The roots of obstacle course racing can be traced back to ancient military training practices, where soldiers underwent physical conditioning and obstacle courses to prepare for combat. However, modern OCR as a competitive sport began to take shape in the late 20th and early 21st centuries. The first major OCR events emerged from the fitness and adventure racing communities, with early examples including the Tough Mudder, which was founded in 2010, and Spartan Race, which began in 2010 as well. These events popularized the format by introducing a mix of endurance running and challenging physical obstacles, drawing inspiration from both military training and adventure sports.

The sport quickly gained popularity, expanding globally and leading to the establishment of numerous OCR organizations and competitions. The growth of OCR has been fuelled by its appeal to a broad range of participants, from elite athletes to recreational fitness enthusiasts, and its focus on both individual achievement and team-based challenges.

One of the early notable obstacle course race examples is the Spartan Death Race, first held in 2007. This event is renowned for its gruelling format, which combines endurance running with extreme physical and mental challenges, often spanning 24 hours or more. Participants face a series of unknown obstacles and tasks, which are revealed only during the race, adding an element of unpredictability and requiring both physical resilience and mental fortitude. Another significant event is the Tough Mudder, which introduced long-distance obstacle courses with challenging obstacles and muddy conditions. These early long endurance races set a high bar for the sport, establishing benchmarks for distance, difficulty, and the integration of obstacles, and inspiring similar events to happen worldwide.

Obstacle course races have become increasingly demanding and complex due to advancements in obstacle design, race formats, and participant expectations. Modern races often feature longer courses with more intricate and challenging obstacles, reflecting the sport's evolution towards greater difficulty and variety. Advances in technology and materials have led to the creation of more innovative and physically demanding obstacles, such as high-altitude rope climbs, complex cargo nets, and challenging mud and water elements. Race formats have also evolved, with events incorporating multi-lap courses, ultra-endurance formats, and themed challenges that test different aspects of physical fitness and mental toughness.

The difficulty of an obstacle course race is determined by a combination of physical, technical, and psychological factors. Physically, participants must manage challenges, from running over long distances to tackling demanding obstacles. The technical aspects of the race involve mastering various obstacles, which may include climbing, crawling, swinging, and carrying heavy loads, each requiring specific skills and techniques. Environmental factors, such as weather conditions, muddy or wet terrain, and temperature extremes, can further complicate the race, adding to the physical and mental demands. Here are what I believe to be the world's toughest obstacle course races.

SPARTAN DEATH RACE

- **Location**.. Vermont (United States)
- **Time of year**.............................. June
- **Approximate distance**................. 70 hours
- **Average time to finish**................ 70 hours
- **Average number of entries**.......... 200 – 300 participants
- **Average cost to enter**.................. $400 – $700
- **Year it started**............................ 2005
- **Support offered**.......................... Semi-supported

The Spartan Death Race, founded in 2005, is known as one of the most extreme endurance events on the planet. Set in the challenging terrains of Vermont, the race was designed to push participants to their physical and mental limits. It emerged from the desire to create an endurance race that differed radically from mainstream marathons and triathlons, focusing instead on the unpredictability of tasks and the grit needed to overcome them.

The course of the Spartan Death Race is intentionally left vague and mysterious to participants. The race can include extreme tasks such as heavy lifting, hiking, chopping wood, building structures, or even memorizing Bible verses. The course is set in the Green Mountains, which adds environmental challenges like cold streams, muddy paths, and steep rocky ascents. The unpredictable nature of the tasks, combined with sleep deprivation and the psychological stress of constant surprises, contributes to a high dropout rate. This secrecy and physical demand is what makes the Spartan Death Race notoriously difficult.

To enter the Spartan Death Race, participants must demonstrate a proven track record of endurance. This can include experience in other endurance events, adventure races, or significant athletic achievements. Potential racers must apply and sometimes complete a questionnaire or essay explaining why they believe they are capable of finishing the race. The organizers look for individuals who have a strong mental game and are capable of enduring extreme stress, physical exhaustion, and unpredictable challenges.

You can find more info about the Spartan Death race on their official website:
https://peakraces.com/spartan-death-race/

SPARTAN AGOGE

- **Location**.. Varies each year
- **Time of year**................................... Varies depending on location
- **Approximate distance**.................. 60 hours (as far as possible)
- **Average time to finish**.................. 60 hours
- **Average number of entries**........... 100 participants
- **Average cost to enter**..................... $500 – $800
- **Year it started**............................... 2016
- **Support offered**............................ Supported

The Spartan Agoge is an extreme endurance event designed by Spartan Race, the organization famous for its obstacle course races. Named after the rigorous education and training regimen used in ancient Sparta, the Agoge is intended to test not just physical stamina but also mental toughness, leadership qualities, and teamwork skills. Initiated in 2016, the event draws on historical and mythological elements to create a transformative experience that pushes participants to their limits and beyond.

Unlike traditional races, the Spartan Agoge is not measured by distance but by the duration and variety of challenges over a continuous 60-hour period. The course typically involves natural and man-made obstacles, navigation challenges, survival skills, heavy lifting, and team-based tasks in a remote environment. The event is structured to include not only physical tasks but also intellectual challenges, including problem-solving tasks and leadership exercises. This combination makes the Agoge particularly demanding, as it requires a well-rounded set of capabilities and a high level of resilience.

Entry into the Spartan Agoge requires more than just physical fitness, applicants must demonstrate a background in endurance events or Spartan Races and show a capacity for leadership and teamwork. The application process includes submitting a detailed resume of physical and possibly military or adventure-related experiences. Participants are also encouraged to have completed Spartan's Hurricane Heat or similar endurance events as a prerequisite.

You can find more details about the Spartan Agoge on their official website: https://race.spartan.com/en/race/agoge

WORLD TOUGHEST MUDDER

- **Location**............................... Varies each year
- **Time of year**........................... November
- **Approximate distance**................. 24 hours (as many laps as possible)
- **Average time to finish**............... 24 hours
- **Average number of entries**.......... 1500 participants
- **Average cost to enter**................. $450 – $550
- **Year it started**......................... 2011
- **Support offered**....................... Supported

World's Toughest Mudder (WTM) is the culminating event of the Tough Mudder series, an extreme sports company that hosts obstacle and mud races. Introduced in 2011, WTM was designed to push the boundaries of endurance in obstacle course racing. This 24 hour challenge attracts some of the most hardened endurance athletes from around the globe who come to test their physical limits against some of the most challenging obstacles and harsh racing conditions.

The World's Toughest Mudder course is a brutal 5 mile circuit filled with innovative obstacles, which participants attempt to complete as many times as possible within a 24 hour period. The course includes a mix of physically demanding obstacles such as Funky Monkey, Arctic Enema, and Electroshock Therapy. The race takes place regardless of weather conditions, often adding mud, cold, or heat into the mix, further increasing the difficulty. The 24 hour format tests not only physical stamina but also strategic pacing and teamwork making it one of the most challenging endurance races in the world.

Entry to World's Toughest Mudder is open to anyone willing to accept the challenge. However, to compete for prizes, participants must qualify by completing a Tough Mudder Classic event in the top 5% of finishers or by meeting performance standards in other specified Tough Mudder events throughout the year.

You can find info about the Worlds Toughest Mudder on their official website:
https://toughmudder.co.uk/events/worlds-toughest-mudder/

IRON VIKING

- **Location**.................................... Various (Germany, Netherlands, Scandanavia)
- **Time of year**.............................. Varies depending on location
- **Approximate distance**................. 42km (26.2 mile)
- **Average time to finish**................ 5 – 7 hours
- **Average number of entries**.......... 1000 participants
- **Average cost to enter**.................. $751
- **Year it started**........................... 2010
- **Support offered**......................... Supported

The Iron Viking is considered one of the most challenging events in the Strong Viking obstacle race series, known for pushing physical boundaries. This series, inspired by Viking culture and the historical toughness of Viking warriors, aims to create an environment where participants can test their endurance, strength, and resilience. The Iron Viking specifically offers a marathon-length obstacle course, which is designed to be the ultimate test within the series.

The 42km course of the Iron Viking is laden with over 100 obstacles that challenge every aspect of physical fitness from strength, endurance and agility. Obstacles include mud pits, water crossings, high walls, heavy carries, and rope climbs. Set in rugged terrains that may traverse forested areas, muddy fields, and water bodies, the race is designed to simulate extreme conditions that might have been faced by ancient Viking warriors. The sheer length of the race, combined with the complexity and variety of obstacles, makes completing the Iron Viking a notable achievement.

To enter the Iron Viking, participants must be at least 18 years old and in good physical health. While no specific qualification is required, it is highly recommended that participants train extensively, focusing on cardio, strength training, and obstacle-specific techniques. Participants are also advised to have experience in shorter obstacle course races before attempting the Iron Viking due to its extreme demands.

You can find more details about the Iron Viking race on their official website:
https://strongviking.com/en

ADVENTURE RACING

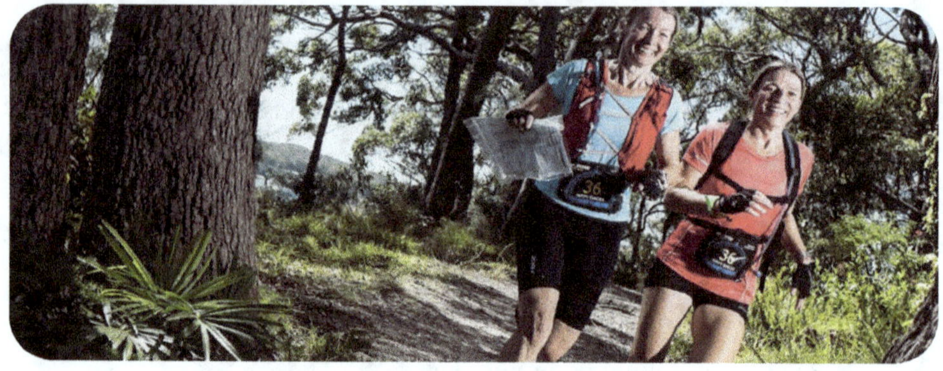

Adventure racing is a demanding endurance sport that combines several outdoor disciplines into a single race, typically including activities such as running, cycling, kayaking, and orienteering. These races are designed to test athletes' versatility and endurance across differing terrains and environments. Participants navigate through varied landscapes, often over long distances and extended periods, using a mix of physical skills and strategic planning. Races are generally non-stop, requiring competitors to transition seamlessly between disciplines. Adventure multisport races can range from short, multi-hour sprints to extended, multi-day expeditions that cover hundreds of miles. The integration of different sports within a single race adds complexity, requiring athletes to train and perform at a high level in multiple disciplines while managing the challenges posed by unpredictable weather and terrain.

The origins of adventure racing can be traced back to the early 20th century, with the rise of expeditionary and military training activities that combined various outdoor skills. However, the sport as it is known today began to take shape in the 1980s and 1990s, when adventure races began gaining popularity as organised events. The Eco-Challenge, founded in 1995 by Mark Burnett, was one of the first major international adventure races, featuring teams competing in a multi-day format across diverse terrains, including mountains, rivers, and jungles. This event helped to popularise the concept of adventure multisport racing and set a high standard for race organization and difficulty. Since then, the sport has evolved with the establishment of numerous adventure racing series and events worldwide, such as the Adventure Racing World Series (ARWS) and various national and regional competitions.

The development of long endurance races in adventure racing began with the introduction of multi-day events that tested participants physical and mental limits over extended periods. The Eco-Challenge, first held in 1995, was among the earliest and most notable long endurance races in the sport.

ADVENTURE RACING

This race covered several hundred miles over diverse terrains, including trekking, biking, and kayaking segments, and required participants to navigate using maps and compasses. The Eco-Challenge set a benchmark for the length and complexity of adventure races, showcasing the combination of endurance, skill, and planning required for such events. Another significant early event is the Primal Quest, which debuted in 2002 and featured a multi-day race format like the Eco-Challenge.

Adventure races have become increasingly challenging as the sport has evolved, driven by advances in race design, and the growing competitiveness of participants. Modern races often feature more complex and demanding courses, incorporating extreme conditions and diverse terrains, such as high-altitude mountain passes, remote jungles, and icy rivers. Advances in equipment, including lightweight and durable gear for trekking, cycling, and kayaking, have enabled races to push the limits of what is physically and technically possible. Race formats have also evolved, with longer distances, more difficult navigation challenges, and multi-stage events that span several days or even weeks.

The difficulty of adventure multisport races arises from a combination of physical, technical, and psychological challenges. Physically, competitors must endure long periods of exertion across diverse activities and terrains, from intense cycling and kayaking to demanding trekking sections. The technical aspects involve mastering a range of skills, such as map reading, compass navigation, and handling complex equipment, while transitioning smoothly between different sports. Environmental factors, including unpredictable weather, rugged terrain, and extreme temperatures, add additional layers of complexity, requiring participants to adapt their strategies and manage their resources effectively. Psychologically, the races demand mental resilience and strategic thinking, as athletes must cope with fatigue, navigate challenging conditions, and maintain focus under pressure.

PATAGONIAN EXPEDITION RACE

- **Location**.. Chile
- **Time of year**................................... February
- **Approximate distance**................. 800km (497 miles)
- **Average time to finish**................. 7 – 10 days
- **Average number of entries**.......... 20 teams
- **Average cost to enter**.................... $5000 – $6000
- **Year it started**............................. 2004
- **Support offered**............................ Semi-supported

The Patagonia Expedition Race is an annual adventure race known for its extreme challenges and stunning backdrop. Founded in 2004, the event quickly earned a reputation as one of the last wild races, designed to test physical endurance, navigation skills, and strategic thinking. Set in the diverse landscape of Southern Patagonia, this race attracts elite adventure racers from around the world. Its goal is not only to provide a competitive racing platform but also to raise awareness of the environmental issues facing this part of the world.

Each edition of the Patagonia Expedition Race features a unique course that is revealed only months before the event. The race covers various disciplines, including trekking, kayaking, mountain biking, and orienteering, across some of the most challenging terrains on earth. Participants must navigate through dense forests, cross icy rivers, traverse mountain ranges, and paddle along windy fjords. The unpredictable weather of Patagonia, with possible sudden storms and strong winds, further adds to the race's difficulty, testing the teams ability to work under pressure.

To participate in the Patagonia Expedition Race, teams must consist of four members, with at least one member of the opposite sex. All participants must have significant experience in multi-discipline endurance events, proven navigation skills, and wilderness survival. Teams are vetted based on their previous racing histories and physical and technical skills to ensure they are capable of safely navigating the demanding conditions of the race. A detailed application process requires teams to submit resumes of each member, a list of equipment, and an outline of their training regimen.

You can find details about Patagonia Expedition race on their official website: https://www.patagonianexpeditionrace.com/en/

EXPEDITION ALASKA

- **Location**.. Alaska (United States)
- **Time of year**.............................. June/ July
- **Approximate distance**................. 700km (435 miles)
- **Average time to finish**................. 7 – 12 days
- **Average number of entries**.......... 20 – 30 teams
- **Average cost to enter**................... $4000 – $6000
- **Year it started**............................. 2007
- **Support offered**........................... Semi-supported

Expedition Alaska is an adventure race known for its intense challenges, set against the backdrop of Alaska's rugged wilderness. First held in 2016, the event was designed to test the limits of endurance athletes through a combination of trekking, mountain biking, and kayaking. It reflects the spirit of adventure racing by incorporating Alaska's vast and varied landscapes, including mountains, forests, rivers, and lakes. Expedition Alaska was created to provide a unique experience that highlights the extreme conditions and spectacular scenery of the Alaskan terrain.

The Expedition Alaska course is known for its sheer difficulty, encompassing a multi-disciplinary race through some of the most challenging and remote landscapes in the state. The course features significant elevation changes, with steep climbs and descents across mountainous terrain, interspersed with technical sections and river crossings. Participants must navigate through dense forests, alpine meadows, and rugged backcountry, often facing unpredictable weather conditions ranging from heavy rains and cold temperatures to strong winds. The remote nature of the course means that support is limited, and competitors must be highly self-sufficient.

To enter, teams must meet specific entry criteria to ensure they are prepared for the event's extreme challenges. Teams typically consist of two to four members who must demonstrate substantial experience in adventure racing or similar endurance events. This includes previous completions of races involving multiple disciplines, such as long-distance trekking, cycling, and kayaking.

You can find more details about Expedition Alaska on their official website:
https://www.warriorraces.com/expedition-alaska

ADVENTURE RACING WORLD CHAMPIONSHIP

- **Location**...................................... Varies each year
- **Time of year**............................... October
- **Approximate distance**.................. 650km (404 miles)
- **Average time to finish**.................. 5 – 7 days
- **Average number of entries**.......... 50 – 60 teams
- **Average cost to enter**................... $4000 – $5000
- **Year it started**............................ 2001
- **Support offered**.......................... Semi-supported

The Adventure Racing World Championship (ARWC) is the premier event in the sport of adventure racing, hosted annually by the Adventure Racing World Series. Since its beginning in 2001, the ARWC has brought together the world's elite adventure racing teams to compete in a non-stop, multi-day race across some of the most challenging and remote environments on the planet. The event rotates among countries, each offering unique terrains and challenges, making each championship a distinctive and memorable experience.

Each ARWC course is designed to be an ultimate test of endurance and team strategy, integrating various disciplines such as trekking, mountain biking, kayaking, and orienteering. The course covers vast distances and often remote terrain, requiring teams to navigate while managing their physical stamina over several days with little or no sleep. Environmental challenges such as river crossings, mountain ascents, and technical rope work can be compounded by adverse weather conditions, adding to the race's difficulty.

Entry into the ARWC is restricted to qualified teams who have demonstrated their capabilities in the Adventure Racing World Series events held globally throughout the year. Teams must finish in top positions at these qualifying events to earn a spot at the World Championship. Each team is typically composed of four members, including at least one member of the opposite sex, to comply with the rules of the series.

You can find more details about adventure racing WC on their official website: https://arworldseries.com/

LEGEND EXPEDITION RACE

- **Location**.. Varies each year
- **Time of year**.................................. March
- **Approximate distance**................. 600 km (372 miles)
- **Average time to finish**................. 6 – 8 days
- **Average number of entries**.......... 20 – 30 teams (4 members each)
- **Average cost to enter**................... $3000 – $4500 per team
- **Year it started**.............................. N/A
- **Support offered**............................ Semi-supported

PRIMAL QUEST

- **Location**............................... Varies each year
- **Time of year**............................. June
- **Approximate distance**................. 450km (280 miles)
- **Average time to finish**................. 5 – 10 days
- **Average number of entries**.......... 40 – 50 teams (4 members each)
- **Average cost to enter**................... $3500 – $4500
- **Year it started**............................. 2002
- **Support offered**........................... Semi-supported

Primal Quest is one of the most prestigious and challenging expedition adventure races in the world. Founded in 2002, the race quickly became known for its gruelling distance. Designed to test human limits, Primal Quest has attracted elite adventure racers from around the globe, looking to compete in the demanding disciplines of kayaking, trekking, mountain biking, and orienteering. After a hiatus, the race has seen several revivals, each time reintroducing a focus on environmental stewardship and adventure.

Primal Quest courses are known for their epic scale and complexity. Each race is set in a remote wilderness area, incorporating natural obstacles and requiring non-stop navigation over varied terrain. The course includes multiple disciplines that require not only physical endurance but also technical skills such as rock climbing, rappelling, river rafting, and advanced orienteering. The unpredictability of weather and terrain adds to the challenge, as teams must manage their physical and mental resources wisely to navigate for 24 hours a day, across vast distances with significant elevation changes.

To enter Primal Quest, teams must consist of four racers, including at least one member of the opposite sex. All team members must have proven experience in multi-day adventure races or a strong background in various endurance sports. Detailed resumes highlighting each member's skills and experience must be submitted as part of the application process.

You can find more details about the Primal Quest on their official website: https://primalquest.org/

COAST-TO-COAST NEW ZEALAND

- **Location**.. New Zealand
- **Time of year**.................................. February
- **Approximate distance**.................. 243km (151 miles)
- **Average time to finish**.................. 10 – 15 hours
- **Average number of entries**.......... 1000 participants
- **Average cost to enter**................... $1000 – $2000
- **Year it started**.............................. 1983
- **Support offered**............................ Supported

The Coast to Coast is an iconic multi-sport event in New Zealand, renowned worldwide for its challenge and the scenic beauty of its course. Founded in 1983 by Robin Judkins, the race quickly became a benchmark for adventure sports enthusiasts looking to test their endurance across diverse terrains. This event has not only contributed to the local economy by attracting international participants but has also inspired a wider appreciation for the landscapes of New Zealand's South Island.

Spanning the width of New Zealand's South Island, the course includes a 3km run, a 55km cycle, a 33km mountain run, a 15km cycle, a 67km kayak, and a final 70km cycle to the finish line. The route traverses the Southern Alps and involves crossing the challenging Goat Pass during the mountain run, navigating the Waimakariri River in a kayak, and biking across the Canterbury Plains. The diversity of the terrain and the physical demands of switching between disciplines add significant complexity. Weather conditions can also vary dramatically, presenting additional challenges such as river crossings at different water levels and variable wind and temperature conditions.

Entry into the race is open to both individual competitors and teams. Participants must be at least 18 years old and are expected to have proficiency in each discipline to ensure safety, especially in kayaking, where strong river skills are crucial. Prior multi-sport or triathlon experience is highly recommended. All entrants must also demonstrate their ability to swim in open water as part of the safety requirements. Registration can be completed online, and participants are encouraged to register early due to the popularity and limited slots in the race.

You can find details about Coast to coast New Zealand on their official website: https://www.coasttocoast.co.nz/

WILDERNESS TRAVERSE

- **Location**....................................... Canada
- **Time of year**................................. September
- **Approximate distance**................. 150km (93 miles)
- **Average time to finish**................. 30 hours
- **Average number of entries**.......... 60 teams (3 - 4 members each)
- **Average cost to enter**................... $900 – $1200
- **Year it started**.............................. 2010
- **Support offered**........................... Semi-supported

Wilderness Traverse is a 24-hour adventure race that challenges teams to navigate through remote backcountry and rugged environments in Ontario, Canada. Since its beginning in 2010, the race has gained a reputation as one of the premier adventure races in Canada, drawing experienced adventure racers and outdoor enthusiasts who are eager to test their skills in navigation, endurance, and teamwork. The event was created to provide an authentic wilderness experience that pushes teams to their limits while exploring the Canadian landscape.

Each year, Wilderness Traverse offers a new and undisclosed course that can include trekking, mountain biking, and canoeing segments. The exact route and disciplines are revealed to teams only hours before the race starts, adding an element of surprise and requiring on-the-spot strategy planning. The course typically spans over 150km of challenging terrain featuring dense forests, steep hills, rocky outcrops, and waterways. This unpredictability, combined with the need for self-sufficiency and continuous movement for up to 30 hours, makes Wilderness Traverse particularly demanding.

To enter, all team members must be at least 18 years old and should possess skills in navigation and endurance sports. While previous adventure racing experience is highly recommended, newcomers with strong backgrounds in related disciplines such as orienteering, paddling, or mountain biking may also compete. Teams must provide their own gear, including navigation tools, first aid supplies, and appropriate clothing for potentially harsh weather conditions. Registration typically opens several months in advance, and due to the race's popularity and limited entry slots, early registration is advised.

You can find details about the Wilderness Traverse on their official website: https://www.wildernesstraverse.com/

RED BULL DEFIANCE

- **Location**...................................... Wanaka (New Zealand)
- **Time of year**............................... January
- **Approximate distance**................. 150km (93 miles)
- **Average time to finish**................. 12 – 18 hours
- **Average number of entries**.......... 100 – 150 teams (2 members each)
- **Average cost to enter**.................. $1200 – $1500
- **Year it started**............................. 2015
- **Support offered**........................... Supported

Red Bull Defiance is a unique multi-sport race designed to test the endurance, determination, and skill of participants in a team format. Launched in 2015 in Wanaka, New Zealand, the race quickly generated a reputation for its challenging courses and the spectacular natural beauty of its settings. Created with the adventure racer in mind, Red Bull Defiance aims to combine traditional endurance disciplines with the added elements of adventure and strategy, making it a standout event in the global adventure racing calendar.

The course is known for its rigorous and varied terrain, typically including mountain biking, kayaking, and running segments, along with strategic navigational challenges. The Wanaka course, for example, involves traversing rugged landscapes, crossing crystal-clear lakes, and climbing steep mountain trails that require both technical skill and physical strength. The difficulty is amplified by the unpredictable weather conditions, which can change swiftly in mountainous regions, adding an additional layer of difficulty. The race's design, which requires teams to not only race against the clock but also manage their resources and equipment efficiently, adds to the overall challenge and appeal.

Entry is open to teams of two, and participants must be over the age of 18. While the race is designed for athletes with a background in multi-sport or adventure racing, newcomers with strong endurance sports experience are also welcome to register. Teams are expected to be self-sufficient in navigation and have a high level of fitness across multiple disciplines. Entry involves submitting an application that may include details of previous race experience, fitness levels, and reasons for participating, which helps ensure that all competitors are prepared for the physical and technical demands of the event.

You can find more details about Red Bull Defiance on their official website: https://defiance.events/

MOTORSPORT

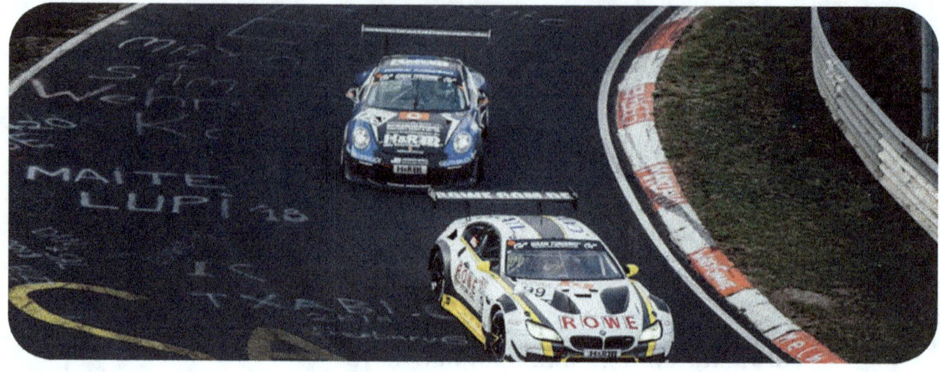

Motorsport racing encompasses a broad spectrum of competitive events where drivers race vehicles designed for speed and agility across various types of tracks and terrains. These events can range from single-seater Formula 1 cars and touring cars to motorcycles and rally vehicles. The races can be conducted on closed-circuit tracks, street circuits, off-road courses, or open roads, each presenting unique challenges and requiring specific skills.

The origins of motorsport racing trace back to the late 19th and early 20th centuries, following the advent of the automobile. The first recorded automobile race took place in 1894 between Paris and Rouen in France, marking the beginning of organized motor racing. This race, known as the Paris-Rouen, was a test of both vehicle reliability and speed. As automotive technology progressed, so did the complexity and popularity of racing. The early 20th century saw the establishment of iconic events like the Monaco Grand Prix (1929) and the 24 Hours of Le Mans (1923), which helped to formalize racing formats and standards. Over the decades, motorsport racing has grown to include a variety of disciplines, from NASCAR and rally racing to endurance and touring car series, each contributing to the sport's history and evolution.

The concept of long endurance races in motorsport began with the early 20th-century events that tested not just speed but also the durability and reliability of vehicles over extended distances. One of the most significant early examples is the 24 Hours of Le Mans, first held in 1923. This race, organized in France, challenged teams to race for 24 hours straight, covering as many laps as possible in that time, and required both driver endurance and vehicle reliability. Another pioneering event was the Mille Miglia, an Italian road race that started in 1927 and covered approximately 1,000 miles of public roads. These races set the stage for modern endurance racing by highlighting the importance of vehicle endurance, team strategy, and driver stamina, paving the way for the development of contemporary endurance events like the World Endurance Championship (WEC) and the Dakar Rally.

Motorsport races have evolved significantly, becoming increasingly challenging due to advancements in technology, changes in race formats, and growing competitive standards. Modern endurance races, such as the 24 Hours of Le Mans and the Dakar Rally, feature sophisticated vehicles with cutting-edge technology, including hybrid powertrains and advanced telemetry systems, which push the limits of speed and efficiency. The complexity of these races has also increased, with the integration of more challenging terrains and environmental conditions, such as extreme weather and off-road obstacles, demanding greater versatility from drivers and vehicles. Additionally, race formats have evolved to include more stages and diverse conditions, such as multi-day rallies and multi-class races, which test the endurance of participants. The continuous innovation in vehicle technology, combined with heightened competition and evolving race conditions, reflects a trend towards more demanding and varied motorsport events.

When selecting what I believe to be the toughest endurance motorsport races, I considered a variety of factors. While technical skill and vehicle performance are essential, endurance racing introduces unique challenges. Drivers must maintain intense focus and peak performance over extended periods, all while managing the physical strain of high G-forces and extreme fatigue. Additionally, environmental factors, such as unpredictable weather or track conditions, amplify the complexity. With these considerations in mind, I've compiled a list of what I believe are the world's most demanding endurance motorsport races. Let's explore them.

AROUND THE WORLD IN 80 DAYS RALLY

- **Location**..................................... Global (starts & finishes in London)
- **Time of year**.............................. August/ September/ October
- **Approximate distance**................. 35,405km (22,000 miles)
- **Average time to finish**................. 80 days
- **Average number of entries**.......... 30 – 40 vehicles
- **Average cost to enter**................... $20,000
- **Year it started**............................. 2002
- **Support offered**........................... Semi-supported

The Around the World in 80 Days Rally is an ambitious motor rally inspired by Jules Verne's classic novel. This rally is not just a test of driving skill but also of endurance and the ability to handle the logistics of an international journey. The event brings together vintage car enthusiasts and travellers, who aspire to do a lap of the world in their classic cars.

Traversing 22,000 miles across four continents, the course challenges participants with a vast array of road conditions, weather climates, and landscapes. Starting from London, competitors drive through Europe into the emptiness of Russia and Mongolia, cross into China, and then ship their vehicles to North America to drive across the United States. The rally then concludes with a final European leg upon returning to London. This route is not only physically demanding due to the long distances and varying road qualities but also logistically complex. Participants must navigate international borders, arrange vehicle shipments, and manage travel in regions where languages vary significantly.

To participate, entrants must own and operate a classic or vintage car that meets specific age and historical authenticity criteria. Typically, vehicles must be at least 20 years old, and often, cars that have historical significance or are of a model that ceased production decades ago are preferred. Prospective participants must submit an application detailing the make and model of their car, their personal and team credentials, and their ability to fund the substantial entry fee and associated costs. Experience in long-distance driving and previous participation in rallies is highly advantageous and often required.

You can find info about the Around the World Rally on their official website: https://80edays.com/

IRON BUTT RALLY

- **Location**... USA
- **Time of year**.................................. June
- **Approximate distance**................. 17,700km (11,000 miles)
- **Average time to finish**.................. 11 days
- **Average number of entries**.......... 100 – 120 participants
- **Average cost to enter**.................... $1500 – $2000
- **Year it started**.............................. 1984
- **Support offered**........................... Supported

The Iron Butt Rally is often referred to as the "World's Toughest Motorcycle Rally," a fitting title for an event that demands riders cover approximately 11,000 miles in just 11 days. Established in 1984 by the Iron Butt Association (IBA), the rally is the pinnacle of long-distance motorcycle riding. The Iron Butt Rally is held every two years and has grown to become one of the most respected and challenging events in the motorcycling world. Unlike traditional races, the Iron Butt Rally emphasizes safe and precise long-distance riding rather than speed, with participants navigating a complex web of checkpoints across the United States and sometimes Canada.

The course is unique in that it changes with every edition, offering a new challenge to participants each time. Riders are not given a fixed route; instead, they receive a list of checkpoints scattered across the country, each with varying point values based on distance and difficulty. Riders must plan their routes strategically to maximize their points while ensuring they complete the required mileage within the 11-day time frame. Participants often ride 1,000 miles or more each day, through all kinds of weather, from scorching heat to torrential rain, and across diverse terrains. Sleep deprivation is a significant challenge, as riders must balance the need for rest with the pressure to maintain their pace.

Entry is highly competitive, with more riders interested in participating than there are available spots. Prospective participants must demonstrate their long-distance riding credentials by completing a series of IBA-certified rides, such as the "SaddleSore 1000" (1,000 miles in 24 hours) or "Bun Burner 1500" (1,500 miles in 36 hours).

You can find further details about Iron Butt Rally on their official website:
https://www.ironbuttrally.net/

PEKING TO PARIS

- **Location**.. Beijing (China) to Paris (France)
- **Time of year**............................... May/ June
- **Approximate distance**................. 14,000km (8,700 miles)
- **Average time to finish**................. 35 days
- **Average number of entries**.......... 100 participants
- **Average cost to enter**................... $20,000
- **Year it started**............................. 1907
- **Support offered**........................... Semi-supported

The Peking to Paris Motor Challenge is one of the most renowned endurance motor rallies in the world. With the first edition in 1907, there were hardly any roads and motoring had only just been born. The challenge was reintroduced in 1997 by the Endurance Rally Association to commemorate the original event and has since been held approximately every three years. The rally is not just a test of driving skill and endurance but also an exploration of the world's most diverse landscapes and cultures, following in the historic tracks of the motorists who made the first journey.

The route from Beijing to Paris is a journey through some of the most remote and challenging terrain on the planet. Participants drive through the Gobi Desert, navigate the traffic of Asian cities, traverse Mongolia, and cross into Europe through Russia and Eastern Europe before finishing in Paris. The course combines rough tracks, paved roads, and everything in between, testing both the mechanical resilience of the vehicles and the endurance of their drivers. The logistical challenges of crossing multiple borders and the need to maintain classic cars over such distances adds layers of complexity to the race.

The Peking to Paris Motor Challenge is open to classic and vintage cars, typically pre-1976. Entrants must demonstrate the reliability of their vehicles through detailed mechanical specifications and previous rally history. A significant part of the entry process involves proving the historical authenticity of the car and its capability to endure such a journey. Drivers are not required to be professional racers, but they must show competent mechanical knowledge. Teams usually consist of at least two members: a driver and a navigator.

You can find further details about Peking to Paris on their official website:
https://www.hero-era.com/rallies/peking-to-paris-2025

DAKAR RALLY

- **Location**.. Saudi Arabia
- **Time of year**.............................. January
- **Approximate distance**................. 8000km (4970 miles)
- **Average time to finish**................. 12 days
- **Average number of entries**.......... 5000 participants
- **Average cost to enter**................... $15,000 – $25,000
- **Year it started**............................. 1978
- **Support offered**........................... Supported

The Dakar Rally is one of the most famous and challenging off-road races in the world, initially starting from Paris (France) to Dakar (Senegal) hence its name. Founded by Thierry Sabine in 1978 after he got lost in the desert during the Abidjan-Nice rally and decided that the desert would be a good location for a regular rally. Due to security threats in Mauritania, the rally was moved to South America in 2009, where it remained until 2019 before moving to Saudi Arabia in 2020. The rally has become a test of endurance and navigation, attracting professional and amateur racers from around the globe.

The Dakar Rally's course through the deserts of Saudi Arabia presents plenty of challenges with the terrain containing sand dunes, rocky canyons, and unpredictable weather conditions. Each stage of the rally offers different terrains and obstacles, requiring competitors to be highly skilled in navigation and vehicle handling. The physical and mental stamina needed to compete in long stages under harsh conditions, along with the logistical challenge of managing supplies and equipment, makes the Dakar not just a race, but a battle against the elements. Additionally, the isolation of the desert environment adds to the difficulty, as assistance can often be hours away.

The Dakar Rally is open to both professional racers and amateurs with sufficient off-road driving experience. Entrants must pass an inspection to ensure their vehicles are equipped to handle the extreme conditions of the rally. This includes safety features, navigation systems, and vehicle durability checks. All participants must also undergo medical checks and safety training sessions. Amateur entrants often participate in "Dakar Challenge" qualifying events, which are held in various locations worldwide and provide a pathway to compete in the main event.

You can find further details about Dakar Rally on their official website:
https://www.dakar.com/en/

AFRICA ECO RACE

- **Location**.. Europe & Africa
- **Time of year**................................. January
- **Approximate distance**................. 6500km (4000 miles)
- **Average time to finish**................ 12 – 14 days
- **Average number of entries**.......... 100 – 150 vehicles
- **Average cost to enter**.................. $12,000 – $25,000
- **Year it started**............................. 2009
- **Support offered**........................... Semi-supported

The Africa Eco Race is a prestigious off-road rally that was established in 2009 as an alternative to the original Paris-Dakar Rally, which moved to South America due to security concerns in Africa. The race aims to maintain the challenge of the original Dakar, with a strong emphasis on eco-friendliness and sustainability. Starting in Europe, often in Monaco, the race covers over 6500km through Morocco, Western Sahara, and Mauritania before finishing in Dakar, Senegal. The event attracts a diverse range of participants, including professional rally teams and amateurs, all drawn by the opportunity to compete in one of the toughest rallies in the world.

The race is divided into daily stages, with each stage presenting its own unique challenges, from navigating through the treacherous dunes of the Sahara to tackling the rocky tracks of the Atlas Mountains. The extreme conditions, including scorching daytime temperatures and cold nights, add to the difficulty. The remoteness of the course also means that participants must be highly self-sufficient, with limited access to outside help in the event of mechanical failure or injury.

The race is open to a wide range of participants competing in various categories such as motorcycles, cars, trucks, and quads. To enter, participants must meet specific criteria, including having a vehicle that meets the race's technical requirements and passing a detailed process. Participants must also have a valid competition license and are encouraged to have prior experience in off-road rallying, given the race's extreme difficulty.

You can find more details about Africa Eco Race on their official website: https://www.africarace.com/en

EAST AFRICAN SAFARI RALLY

- **Location**.................................... Kenya, Tanzania & Uganda
- **Time of year**............................... December
- **Approximate distance**.................. 5000km (3100miles)
- **Average time to finish**................. 9 days
- **Average number of entries**.......... 60 – 70 cars
- **Average cost to enter**.................. $15,000
- **Year it started**............................ 1953
- **Support offered**.......................... Semi-supported

The East African Safari Rally, originally known as the Coronation Safari, was first held in 1953 to celebrate the coronation of Queen Elizabeth II. It quickly evolved into one of the most prestigious rallies in the world, known for its harsh conditions and challenging routes. It became a part of the World Rally Championship in the 1970s but was later excluded due to its difficulty and logistics. In recent years, it has been revived as a classic rally, attracting vintage car enthusiasts who seek to experience the challenge of the original event.

The rally is famed for its challenging course, which covers thousands of kilometers through some of Africa's most diverse terrains. The route traverses dusty and rocky roads, muddy paths during the rainy season, and extends through remote areas with minimal infrastructure. Drivers and teams face extreme weather conditions, from intense heat to torrential rains, which can transform dry riverbeds into impassable routes within hours. The demanding nature of the terrain, combined with the need for navigational skills and vehicle reliability, tests the endurance and skill of even the most experienced rally drivers.

To enter the East African Safari Rally, participants typically need to own a classic or historically significant rally car, generally pre-1986. Entries are evaluated based on the car's historical significance, compliance with safety standards, and suitability for enduring the harsh conditions of the rally. Teams must also provide information about their racing and mechanical experience. Due to the rigorous nature of the rally, a comprehensive understanding of vehicle maintenance and off-road driving is essential for all participants.

You can find details about East African Safari Rally on their official website:
https://eastafricansafarirally.com/

24 HOURS OF LE MANS

- **Location**............................... France
- **Time of year**............................. June
- **Approximate distance**................. 5000km (3100miles)
- **Average time to finish**................. 24 hours
- **Average number of entries**.......... 60 cars
- **Average cost to enter**.................. $100,000
- **Year it started**............................. 1923
- **Support offered**............................ Supported

The 24 Hours of Le Mans is an event held annually at Circuit de la Sarthe in Le Mans, France, is one of the most prestigious automobile races in the world and a cornerstone of the endurance motorsport racing calendar. It was first run in 1923 with the aim of encouraging automotive innovation and testing car reliability over long distances. Over the decades, Le Mans has evolved into a test of endurance that challenges the limits of both car and driver, emphasizing the importance of speed and durability. The race is part of the Triple Crown of Motorsport, which also includes the Indianapolis 500 and the Monaco Grand Prix.

The Circuit de la Sarthe, where the 24 Hours of Le Mans is held, combines public roads and specialised racing tracks, making it one of the longest circuits in the world. The 13.6km circuit is known for its complex corners, high-speed straights, and variable weather conditions, all of which test the cars to their limits. The race runs non-stop for 24 hours, meaning teams must perform under the pressure of continuous day and night racing, managing fatigue and ensuring their vehicles withstand the test of time. Strategic planning, including pit stops for fuel, tires, and repairs, plays a crucial role.

Participation in the 24 Hours of Le Mans requires teams to qualify through a series of events governed by the Automobile Club de l'Ouest (ACO), including the World Endurance Championship. Vehicles must meet strict technical specifications tailored to various racing classes. Teams must also present a competitive driver lineup, often including at least one professional driver. Given the technical and financial demands, entries typically come from established racing teams capable of developing vehicles that meet the standards.

You can find details about the 24 Hours of Le Mans on their official website: https://www.24h-lemans.com/en

IRONDOG

- **Location**.................................... Alaska (United States)
- **Time of year**............................. February
- **Approximate distance**................ 4023km (2500 miles)
- **Average time to finish**................ 7 – 10 days
- **Average number of entries**.......... 25 – 35 participants
- **Average cost to enter**.................. $3000 – $5000
- **Year it started**........................... 1984
- **Support offered**.......................... Semi-supported

Iron Dog is the world's longest and most challenging snowmobile race, held annually across the remote terrain of Alaska. Established in 1984, the race was originally known as the Iron Dog Gold Rush Classic and was intended to test the endurance and skills of snowmobile enthusiasts. Over the years, the Iron Dog has grown in prominence, becoming a premier event in the world of snowmobile racing. The race starts in Big Lake, Alaska, traveling westward to Nome, and then looping back east to finish in Fairbanks. The Iron Dog is not just a race; it's a test of survival, mechanical expertise, and strategic planning.

The course is infamous for its length and the extreme conditions. The route includes frozen rivers, dense forests, mountain ranges, and vast tundra, where temperatures can plummet to -50°F (-45°C) or lower. Riders must navigate through blizzards, whiteouts, and hazardous terrain, often traveling at high speeds while avoiding hidden obstacles like ice ridges and open water. The course is divided into multiple checkpoints, where teams can refuel, make repairs, and rest briefly. However, the vast distances between these checkpoints mean that teams must be self-sufficient, carrying the necessary gear and spare parts to deal with breakdowns or emergencies.

For entry into the race, each team must consist of two riders, and both must have significant experience in long-distance snowmobiling and survival skills in extreme cold. Before the race, all participants must undergo a rigorous technical inspection to ensure their snowmobiles meet the race's stringent safety and performance standards.

You can find further details about the Irondog race on their official website: https://www.irondog.org/

24 HOURS OF DAYTONA

- **Location**.. Florida (United States)
- **Time of year**................................ January
- **Approximate distance**................. 4000km (2500 miles)
- **Average time to finish**................. 24 hours
- **Average number of entries**.......... 50 cars
- **Average cost to enter**.................. N/A
- **Year it started**............................ 1962
- **Support offered**........................... Supported

The 24 Hours of Daytona, officially known as the Rolex 24 at Daytona, is a 24-hour sports car endurance race held annually at Daytona International Speedway in Daytona Beach, Florida. The race started in 1962 as a three-hour event, it has since grown in prestige to become one of the most important races in the IMSA WeatherTech SportsCar Championship and a major event in the international motorsports calendar.

The Daytona International Speedway presents a unique challenge, combining a high-speed tri-oval with a tight and technical infield road course. Totalling 3.56 miles per lap, the layout requires cars to handle high-speed banking turns as well as slower, twistier sections that test braking and handling. The race's duration requires teams to perform under the intense pressure of continuous racing through day and night, in variable weather conditions ranging from cool nights to potentially warm daytime temperatures. Teams must balance speed with mechanical reliability and manage frequent pit stops for fuel, tires, and repairs, all while navigating traffic from other teams on the track.

Entry is governed by the International Motor Sports Association (IMSA). Teams must comply with IMSA regulations, which stipulate various requirements for vehicles competing in different classes. Participants are required to have proper credentials and racing licenses, and teams typically consist of professional drivers or highly experienced amateurs. Teams must also demonstrate financial and logistical capabilities to compete in such a demanding event, including support crews capable of maintaining high-performance racing vehicles over 24 hours.

You can find details about 24 Hours of Daytona on their official website: https://www.imsa.com/events/24-at-daytona/

CAINS QUEST

- **Location**.................................... Canada
- **Time of year**.............................. March
- **Approximate distance**................. 3100km (1926 miles)
- **Average time to finish**................ 7 – 10 days
- **Average number of entries**.......... 30 – 40 teams
- **Average cost to enter**.................. $5000 – $8000
- **Year it started**............................ 2006
- **Support offered**.......................... Semi-supported

Cain's Quest is the longest and most challenging snowmobile endurance race in North America, held every two years in the remote wilderness of Labrador, Canada. Established in 2006, the race was created to showcase the extreme winter conditions and the stunning, yet unforgiving, terrain of Labrador. What started as a local event has quickly grown into an internationally recognized race, attracting teams from around the world.

The Cain's Quest course is renowned for its extreme difficulty, spanning approximately 3100km through the remote and often treacherous terrain of Labrador. The race begins and ends in Labrador City, with the course winding through deep snow, frozen lakes, dense forests, and rugged mountains. Teams must navigate the course using GPS, dealing with sub-zero temperatures that can drop as low as -40°C (-40°F), blizzards, and whiteout conditions. The remote location of the race means that teams are often hundreds of kilometers from the nearest town or support, adding to the challenge. The race is divided into several checkpoints, but the vast distances between them require teams to be self-sufficient, carrying enough fuel, food, and emergency supplies to survive the harsh conditions. The demands of this race often mean participants will be riding a snowmobile for up to 20 hours a day.

Entry into the race requires you to be part of a team. Each team consists of two riders, and both must have significant experience in long-distance snowmobiling and survival skills in extreme winter conditions.

You can find further details about Cains Quest on their official website:
https://cainsquest.com/

BAJA 1000

- **Location**.. Mexico
- **Time of year**.................................. November
- **Approximate distance**................ 1609km (1000 miles)
- **Average time to finish**................ 20 – 30 hours
- **Average number of entries**.......... 250 – 350 participants
- **Average cost to enter**.................. $3000 – $6000
- **Year it started**............................. 1967
- **Support offered**........................... Supported

The Baja 1000 is one of the most legendary off-road races in the world, held annually on Mexico's Baja California Peninsula. First organized in 1967, the race was initially a test of endurance for both vehicles and drivers, quickly earning its reputation as one of the toughest motorsport events on the planet. Over the decades, the Baja 1000 has become a defining event in off-road racing, attracting top competitors from around the world, including professional drivers and even celebrities. The race features a wide variety of vehicle classes, including motorcycles, trucks, buggies, and ATV's.

The route changes each year, alternating between a point-to-point race from Ensenada to La Paz and a loop course that starts and ends in Ensenada. The terrain includes a mix of sandy deserts, rocky mountain trails, dry lake beds, and coastal paths. Drivers must navigate through deep silt beds, sharp rocks, treacherous ravines, and steep ascents, all while contending with extreme heat, dust, and the possibility of mechanical failure. The race runs non-stop, meaning that teams must strategize when to push forward and when to conserve their vehicles and energy. Many sections of the course are remote and inaccessible, increasing the risk and difficulty of providing assistance in case of a breakdown or accident.

Entry is open to a wide range of participants, from professional teams to amateur racers, but it requires serious preparation and commitment. Beyond the entry fee, teams must be prepared for significant logistical and financial commitments, including vehicle preparation, support crews, and spare parts. The race requires a strong support team to manage fuel stops, repairs, and rider changes, as well as to provide food and rest when needed.

You can find more details about Baja 1000 on their official website: https://score-international.com/

MILLE MIGLIA

- **Location**............................... Italy
- **Time of year**............................. May
- **Approximate distance**................. 1600km (1000 miles)
- **Average time to finish**................. 4 days
- **Average number of entries**.......... 400 cars
- **Average cost to enter**.................. $7000
- **Year it started**.......................... 1927
- **Support offered**......................... Semi-supported

The Mille Miglia, often referred to as "the most beautiful race in the world," is a historic car rally that initially ran as a speed race from 1927 to 1957. The race was discontinued due to safety concerns but was revived in 1977 as a regularity rally for classic and vintage cars, celebrating the heritage and romanticism of early motor racing. The modern version of the Mille Miglia is not only a competitive event but also a rolling museum of automotive history, attracting car enthusiasts and collectors from around the globe who come to experience Italy's landscapes and towns.

The Mille Miglia route covers approximately 1600 kilometers from Brescia to Rome and back, with a mix of fast straights, winding country roads, and mountain passes. The difficulty lies not just in the physical driving but in the precision required for regularity racing, where consistency and adherence to strict timing are more important than speed. Navigating this historic course requires significant skill, especially given the unpredictable Italian weather and the complexities of managing vintage machinery over such distances. Additionally, the rally passes through numerous small towns, where narrow streets and crowds add to the driving challenge.

Entry into the Mille Miglia is highly selective, restricted to cars that would have been eligible for the original races held between 1927 and 1957. Applicants must submit detailed documentation proving the authenticity and historical value of their vehicle. Additionally, due to the rally's prestigious nature and the physical demands of the event, drivers are often required to demonstrate previous experience in classic car rallies or possess significant skills in handling vintage automobiles in races. The selection process is rigorous, emphasizing the preservation of the rally's history and the safety of participants.

You can find further details about the Mille Miglia on their official website:
https://1000miglia.it/en/

RUCKING

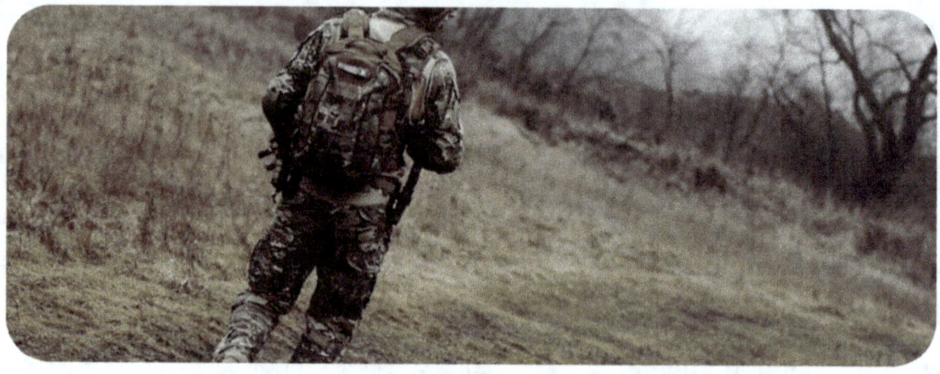

Rucking is a form of endurance training or racing where participants walk or run while carrying a weighted backpack, often called a rucksack. These races challenge competitors to traverse various terrains, such as trails and roads all while bearing the additional weight. The races can vary in distance from short sprints to long, multi-day events, and the weight carried in the rucksack can be a crucial factor in the challenge. These events are popular among military personnel, outdoor enthusiasts, and athletes looking for a rigorous test of their stamina and resilience.

The origins of rucking can be traced back to military training, where soldiers were required to carry heavy loads over long distances as part of their physical conditioning and operational readiness. The term "ruck" comes from the military slang for a backpack or rucksack. The practice of rucking has evolved from these military roots into a broader fitness and competitive discipline. In recent years, rucking has gained popularity outside of military contexts, becoming a staple in fitness challenges. The shift towards civilian rucking began as athletes and fitness enthusiasts sought new ways to push their limits and test their endurance.

The concept of long endurance rucking races began to formalize in the early 2000s. One of the earliest and most notable events in this category was the GoRuck Challenge, which started in 2010. This event was inspired by the military's rigorous training methods and aimed to bring the rucking experience to a civilian audience. The GoRuck Challenge, and similar events, combined long-distance rucking with elements of team-building, tactical training, and obstacle courses, making it a comprehensive endurance test. These early races often featured distances of 12 to 20 miles with weight requirements typically ranging from 20 to 30 pounds. The introduction of these long endurance events helped establish rucking as a competitive and fitness-oriented activity, paving the way for more specialized and varied rucking races.

Rucking races have evolved significantly since their inception, becoming increasingly demanding and diverse in their formats. Modern rucking events often include additional elements beyond simple long-distance marching with weight. Organizers have incorporated obstacles, navigational challenges, and team-based tasks to enhance the difficulty and engagement of the races. The weight requirements have also become more rigorous, with some races mandating heavier loads or longer distances. Moreover, races are now being held in more challenging environments, such as extreme weather conditions or rugged terrains, adding another layer of difficulty. The integration of tactical training aspects, inspired by military practices, and the rise of competitive rucking leagues have further pushed the boundaries of what these races entail, making them a true test of endurance, strength, and mental toughness.

The difficulty of a rucking race is influenced by several key factors, each contributing to the overall challenge. Firstly, the weight carried in the rucksack plays a significant role; heavier loads increase the physical strain on participants and can lead to fatigue and discomfort especially over sustained distances. Secondly, the terrain and environmental conditions of the race can greatly affect difficulty. Courses that include uneven or steep terrain demand greater physical effort and can heighten the risk of injury. Weather conditions, such as extreme heat, cold, or rain, also add to the challenge by affecting both the physical and mental endurance of competitors. The duration of the race, combined with the weight and environmental factors, tests participants' ability to maintain stamina and focus over extended periods. It's for this reason, I believe these are the toughest rucking races in the world.

NIJMEGEN MARCHES

- **Location**............................... Netherlands
- **Time of year**.............................. July
- **Approximate distance**................. 200km (124 miles)
- **Average time to finish**................ 4 days
- **Average number of entries**.......... 50,000 participants
- **Average cost to enter**.................. $100
- **Year it started**............................ 1909
- **Support offered**.......................... Supported

The International Four Days Marches Nijmegen, commonly referred to as the "Vierdaagse," is the largest multiple day marching event in the world. It began in 1909 and has been held annually in Nijmegen, Netherlands, attracting participants from all over the globe. The event was initially a military exercise but has evolved into a popular civilian marching festival, celebrating physical fitness and international friendship. It includes a wide range of participants, from military teams to civilian walkers of all ages.

The challenge of the Four Days Marches lies not in speed but in endurance. Participants walk substantial distances (30, 40, or 50km) each day for four consecutive days, covering a variety of terrains around Nijmegen, including city streets, wooded paths, and open countryside. The July timing often means marchers face high temperatures, adding to the physical strain. The cumulative effect of multiple days of long-distance walking tests participants' stamina, foot care, and overall physical conditioning, making this much more than a simple walking event.

The Vierdaagse is open to both military and civilian participants. Civilians can choose their distance based on age and gender guidelines, while military participants often carry a rucksack weighing at least 10kg as part of their challenge. There are no qualification requirements beyond the ability to complete the chosen distance, but registration is capped and often fills up quickly due to the event's popularity. Prospective walkers must register during the official entry period, typically a few months before the event, and often participate as part of a group or club, though individual entries are also accepted.

You can find details about the Nijmegen marches on their official website: https://www.4daagse.nl/en

GORUCK SELECTION

- **Location**.. United States
- **Time of year**.................................. Held twice per year
- **Approximate distance**.................. 128km (80 miles)
- **Average time to finish**.................. 48 hours
- **Average number of entries**........... 100 – 150 participants
- **Average cost to enter**.................... $400
- **Year it started**.............................. 2010
- **Support offered**............................. Supported

GORUCK Selection is an extreme endurance event designed to simulate the U.S. Army Special Forces Assessment and Selection course. It was started in 2010 by Jason McCarthy, a former Green Beret, to test the physical and mental resilience of participants in a controlled, yet very demanding environment. Unlike other GORUCK events which encourage team dynamics and leadership, Selection is an individual event where the completion rates are exceedingly low.

The course for GORUCK Selection is shrouded in secrecy until the event begins, adding an element of unpredictability and stress. The challenges are continuous over 48 hours with no scheduled sleep, the tasks such as rucking with weight, navigation, PT (physical training) tests, and mental toughness scenarios under stressful conditions become even more challenging. The event is run by cadre who are mostly former Special Forces, who ensure the standards are strictly military-grade. The unpredictability of tasks, combined with the physical demand and sleep deprivation, makes this one of the hardest endurance tests comparable to actual military selection courses.

Entry into GORUCK Selection requires participants to be in excellent physical condition with preparation in endurance and strength training. Prior experience in GORUCK challenges or similar endurance events is highly recommended. Participants must also pass a physical fitness test at the beginning of the event, which includes a certain number of push-ups, sit-ups, and a timed run, all conducted under the watchful eye of the cadre to ensure readiness for the upcoming challenges.

You can find further details about GoRuck Selection on their official website:
https://www.goruck.com/pages/goruck-selection

CATERAN YOMP

- **Location**...................................... United Kingdom
- **Time of year**............................. June
- **Approximate distance**................. 87km (54 miles)
- **Average time to finish**................ 24 – 30 hours
- **Average number of entries**.......... 800 – 1000 participants
- **Average cost to enter**................... $60 – $100
- **Year it started**............................. 2010
- **Support offered**........................... Supported

The Cateran Yomp is a celebrated endurance event held annually in Scotland, renowned for its challenging routes and the stunning backdrop of the Scottish Highlands. Established in 2010, the Yomp was created by the Army Benevolent Fund, now known as ABF The Soldiers' Charity, as a means of raising funds for soldiers, veterans, and their families. The Yomp has quickly grown in popularity, drawing participants from various backgrounds who seek to test their endurance while supporting a noble cause.

The Cateran Yomp features three distinct routes, each designed to test different levels of endurance: 22 miles, 36 miles, and 54 miles. The course traverses the Cateran Trail, a scenic yet challenging path that winds through the terrain of Perthshire and Angus. Participants face a variety of obstacles, including steep ascents, rocky paths, and moorland bogs. The combination of the diverse terrain, unpredictable weather, and the sheer distance of the longest route makes the Cateran Yomp a formidable challenge that tests every aspect of an endurance athlete's capability.

To enter there are no stringent qualification requirements for the shorter 22-mile and 36-mile routes, making them accessible to a broader range of participants, including beginners and those with varying levels of fitness. However, the 54-mile route is particularly demanding and typically attracts more experienced walkers and runners. While no formal qualification is required, participants are strongly encouraged to have prior experience in long-distance walking or running to handle the physical demands of the longer course.

You can find further details about the Cateran Yomp on their official website: https://events.armybenevolentfund.org/cateranyomp

WINTER DEATH RACE

- **Location**.. Vermont (United States)
- **Time of year**................................. June
- **Approximate distance**................. 65km (40 miles)
- **Average time to finish**................. 72 hours
- **Average number of entries**.......... 100 – 200 participants
- **Average cost to enter**................... $400 – $900
- **Year it started**.............................. 2005
- **Support offered**........................... Semi-supported

The Spartan Winter Death Race is an extreme endurance event designed to push participants to their mental and physical limits. Held annually in the town of Pittsfield, Vermont, this race was developed as a winter counterpart to the original Death Race, founded in 2005. The Winter Death Race challenges participants with unforeseen tasks and obstacles in harsh winter conditions. The race's motto, "You May Die," underscores its severity and the high level of commitment required to even consider participating.

Set in the winter landscape of Vermont, the course for the Spartan Winter Death Race offers no mercy. Participants may find themselves chopping wood for hours, trekking through waist-deep snow, submerging in icy waters, or solving complex puzzles after physical exhaustion. The race is designed to induce fatigue, hypothermia, and mental exhaustion, simulating survival conditions in extreme cold. The unpredictability of the tasks, combined with the weather conditions and the race's continuous, multi-day format, makes completing the Winter Death Race one of the toughest feats in endurance sports.

Entry into the Spartan Winter Death Race is intentionally made difficult to ensure that only the most determined and prepared individuals participate. Prospective racers must apply by detailing their physical conditioning, endurance event history and reasons for wanting to compete in such a demanding event. Previous experience in endurance and survival events is highly recommended. Participants must also sign a waiver acknowledging the risks and the potential for physical and mental stress.

You can find details about the Winter Death Race on their official website: https://peakraces.com/winter-death-race/

BATAAN MEMORIAL DEATH MARCH

- **Location**.. New Mexico (United States)
- **Time of year**............................... March
- **Approximate distance**................. 42km (26.2 miles)
- **Average time to finish**................ 5 – 8 hours
- **Average number of entries**.......... 8000 participants
- **Average cost to enter**................... $150
- **Year it started**.............................. 1989
- **Support offered**............................ Supported

The Bataan Memorial Death March is a challenging annual march that takes place at the White Sands Missile Range in New Mexico. It was established in 1989 to honour the heroic service members who defended the Philippine Islands during World War II, suffering through harsh conditions in the infamous 1942 Bataan Death March. The event attracts military and civilian participants from all over the world, who march to remember the sacrifices of these soldiers.

The course of the Bataan Memorial Death March is renowned for its gruelling conditions, traversing the hilly terrain of the White Sands Missile Range. The full marathon distance challenges participants with a mix of paved roads and sandy trails, with significant elevation changes. Environmental factors play a huge role, as the march is conducted in a desert setting with possible extreme temperature shifts from morning to midday.

The Bataan Memorial Death March is open to participants of all fitness levels and ages, with categories for military and civilians alike. There are no specific physical prerequisites, but due to the demanding nature of the course, it is highly recommended that individuals train adequately. Participants can choose to march in heavy division (35lbs backpack) or light division (without a backpack). Military participants often march in formation and full gear.

You can find info about Bataan Memorial Death March on their official website:
https://bataanmarch.com/

TOUGH RUCK BOSTON

- **Location**..................................... Massachusetts (United States)
- **Time of year**............................... April
- **Approximate distance**................ 42km (26.2 miles)
- **Average time to finish**................ 5 – 7 hours
- **Average number of entries**.......... 1000 participants
- **Average cost to enter**................... $150
- **Year it started**............................ 2017
- **Support offered**.......................... Supported

Tough Ruck Boston is organized by the Military Friends Foundation in partnership with the Boston Athletic Association and the National Park Service. The event honours military personnel and first responders who have died in the line of duty, with participants carrying rucksacks filled with weight to mimic those in military service. The event has grown significantly since its beginning, becoming an official part of the Boston Marathon events to accommodate more participants and provide a more historic route.

The Tough Ruck Boston course follows the historic Battle Road Trail, famous for its role in the early stages of the American Revolutionary War. The trail presents a variety of challenging terrains, including rough paths, wooded sections, and slight hills. The event takes place regardless of weather conditions, which can vary dramatically in New England in April, potentially adding rain, mud, or even residual snow to the mix.

Entry into Tough Ruck Boston is open to both military personnel and civilians. Participants must register in advance and are encouraged to fundraise for the Military Friends Foundation. The weight classes for the rucksacks are based on the participant's choice: 15lbs for participants 150lbs and under (light), 25lbs for those over 150lbs (medium), and 35lbs for the competitive Heavy Division. All participants must adhere to safety guidelines, including wearing a high-visibility vest and carrying hydration and emergency contact information.

You can find details about Tough Ruck Boston on their official website:
https://www.toughruck.org/

HORSE RACING

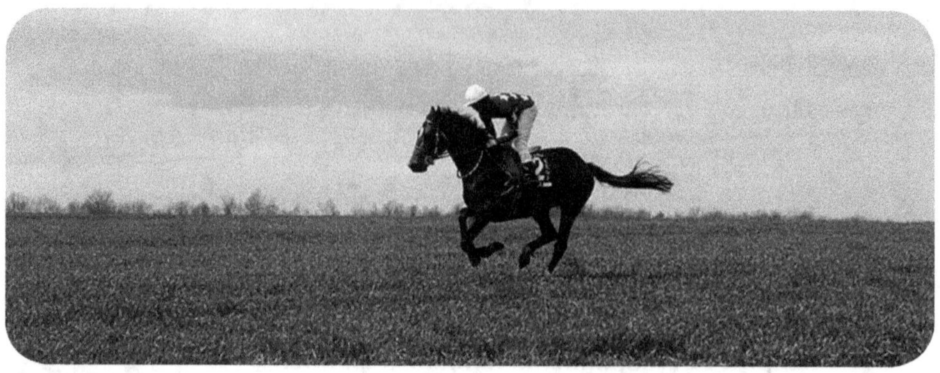

Horse racing is a time-honoured sport that involves horses racing against each other on a defined route, with the objective of reaching the finish line first. In modern horse racing, events can range from local meets to prestigious international races, each governed by specific rules and regulations.

Horse racing's origins trace back to ancient civilizations, where it was a popular pastime among the Greeks, Romans, and Egyptians. Early forms of the sport were often linked to chariot races and mounted contests. By the medieval period, horse racing had evolved into more organized events, with formal races held during festivals and royal gatherings. The sport gained significant traction in the 17th century with the establishment of the Jockey Club in England, which standardized rules and promoted the growth of racing as a regulated sport. The 19th century saw the expansion of horse racing across the globe, with notable events such as the Kentucky Derby in the United States and the Melbourne Cup in Australia becoming cornerstones of the sport. Over the centuries, horse racing has evolved from informal contests into a major global industry.

The concept of long-distance horse racing, or endurance racing, has roots that extend back to ancient times. However, it was during the 19th century that the sport began to formalize and gain recognition. One of the earliest notable long-distance races was the "Century Stakes" held in New York in the early 1800s, featuring distances of around 1.5 miles. As the sport progressed, races of 3 miles or more became increasingly common, pushing the limits of both horse and rider. Endurance racing was also popularized in the military, where long rides and marches tested the stamina and resilience of horses in practical settings. The development of endurance races was crucial in highlighting the horses' ability to maintain speed over extended periods, leading to the establishment of modern long-distance events such as the Tevis Cup, which challenges horse and rider to navigate over 100 miles.

Modern horse racing has seen a significant evolution in demands of its races. Advances in breeding and training have resulted in horses that are faster, more resilient, and capable of handling a variety of racing conditions. The integration of technology has further pushed the boundaries, with sophisticated data analytics and biomechanics providing insights into performance and enhancing training regimens for the horses and riders. Races are now more physically demanding due to the increased competitiveness and the incorporation of challenging track conditions. In recent years, the rules and regulations concerning horse welfare have become significantly stricter. As a result, even in the most challenging races, veterinarians and equestrian professionals are always present, ensuring that the well-being of the horses is a top priority.

Several factors contribute to the difficulty of a horse race. The distance of the race is a primary factor, with longer distances requiring sustained stamina and strategy. Track conditions also play a crucial role; muddy, uneven, or challenging surfaces can significantly impact performance. The competition level is another significant aspect, as highly competitive fields mean that each race is a test of speed and skill against other top-tier contenders. Additionally, weather conditions can make races more challenging, with extreme heat, cold, or rain affecting both the horses and riders ability to perform.

MONGOL DERBY

- **Location**..................................... Mongolia
- **Time of year**............................. August
- **Approximate distance**................. 1000km (621 miles)
- **Average time to finish**................ 7 – 10 days
- **Average number of entries**.......... 40 – 45 participants
- **Average cost to enter**................... $14,000 – $15,000
- **Year it started**............................. 2009
- **Support offered**........................... Semi-supported

The Mongol Derby is renowned as the longest horse race in the world. Established in 2009, the race was created to honour and recreate the ancient postal system of Genghis Khan, who established a vast network of horse stations that allowed riders to cover incredible distances with unparalleled speed and efficiency. This modern-day endurance race draws participants from around the globe, each eager to test their limits against the harsh conditions of Mongolia's wilderness.

The course is divided into 25 - 40km segments, each corresponding to a traditional "urtuu" or horse station, where riders must change horses. Competitors ride semi-wild Mongolian horses, known for their toughness and resilience but also for their unpredictable nature. The race requires riders to navigate without marked trails, relying solely on GPS and their instincts, which adds to the challenge. Weather conditions can vary drastically, with scorching heat during the day and freezing temperatures at night. The terrain itself is treacherous, with riders facing everything from deep river crossings to steep mountain passes while riding up to 14 hours a day.

Entry into the Mongol Derby is highly competitive, with only 40 - 45 spots available each year. Prospective participants must demonstrate significant riding experience, particularly in long-distance and endurance riding. The race organisers seek riders who not only have the technical skills to handle semi-wild horses but also the physical and mental resilience to endure the race conditions. Applicants must provide a detailed riding resume and may be required to undergo an interview process to assess their suitability for the race.

You can find details about the Mongol Derby on their official website: https://equestrianists.com/mongol-derby/

SHAHZADA MEMORIAL ENDURANCE TEST

- **Location**.................................... Australia
- **Time of year**............................... August
- **Approximate distance**................. 400km (250 miles)
- **Average time to finish**............... 5 days
- **Average number of entries**.......... 60 – 80 participants
- **Average cost to enter**.................. $500 – $700
- **Year it started**............................ 1981
- **Support offered**........................... Semi-supported

The Shahzada Memorial Endurance Test is one of Australia's most revered endurance horse races, held annually in the historic village of St. Albans, New South Wales. Established in 1981, the race was created to honour the legendary Arabian stallion Shahzada, who was known for his extraordinary endurance and speed. The event quickly gained a reputation as one of the most challenging endurance tests in the equestrian world, attracting riders to showcasing the stamina of their horses. Over the years, Shahzada has become a cornerstone of the Australian endurance riding community, celebrated not just as a race, but as a gathering of dedicated riders who share a deep respect for the sport and the horses that make it possible.

The race takes place in the hilly and often treacherous terrain surrounding St. Albans, with riders navigating steep ascents, rocky trails, and dense forests. The course is designed to test the limits of both horse and rider, with daily stages ranging from 70 – 100km. The race is also held in late August, when weather conditions can vary widely, adding another layer of difficulty.

Entry into the race is open to experienced endurance riders who have a proven track record in long-distance events. To qualify, riders must have completed several endurance rides, including at least one 160km (100 mile) event. Horses must also meet strict health and conditioning standards, as they will be subjected to rigorous veterinary checks before, during, and after each stage of the race.

You can find info about the Shahzada Memorial Test on their official website: https://www.shahzada400.com/

THE TEVIS CUP

- **Location**.. California (United States)
- **Time of year**.................................. July
- **Approximate distance**.................. 160km (100 miles)
- **Average time to finish**.................. 12 – 24 hours
- **Average number of entries**........... 150 – 200 participants
- **Average cost to enter**.................... $300 – $500
- **Year it started**............................... 1955
- **Support offered**............................. Supported

The Tevis Cup is a prestigious horse race that takes place annually in California. Established in 1955, it was inspired by the historic Tevis Cup, which retraced the original 100-mile ride from the 19th century, when it was used to transport cattle between the Sacramento Valley and the mining camps in Sierra Nevada. Officially known as the Tevis Cup 100-Mile Endurance Ride, this race is a test of stamina and partnership between horse and rider. The event is hosted by the Western States Trail Foundation and is celebrated for its rich history.

The Tevis Cup covers diverse terrain of the Western States Trail in California's Sierra Nevada Mountains. The course begins in the town of Auburn and ends at the end of the trail in the town of Foresthill. It features significant elevation changes, with riders ascending and descending over 18,000 feet (5,500 meters) throughout the race. The trail includes a variety of challenging conditions, such as steep climbs, rocky paths, and narrow, technical sections, which test the endurance and agility of both horse and rider. The race typically takes place in mid-July, and participants must contend with extreme temperatures that can range from scorching heat to cooler mountain conditions. Additionally, the race is run in a single day, requiring riders to manage their horse's stamina, hydration, and nutrition over an extended period.

Entering the Tevis Cup requires specific criteria. Competitors must have completed a qualifying ride prior to the Tevis Cup, typically including a minimum of 50 miles at a competitive pace. Additionally, participants must be members of the American Endurance Ride Conference (AERC) or an equivalent international organization. Both horse and rider must also pass a veterinary examination before the race to ensure they are fit for the demanding course.

You can find further information about the Tevis Cup on their official website: https://teviscup.org/

CHAPTER 2 – AIR SPORTS

In Chapter 2, we explore some of the most challenging air sports in the world, where athletes push the boundaries of what activities can be included in a race. These sports demand not only skill and strategy but also extraordinary mental and physical endurance to battle against the elements while airbourne. Paragliding, in particular, is far more than simply gliding through the air; it's a true test of endurance, precision, and the pilot's ability to harness the invisible forces of nature. Pilots often spend hours suspended in the air, relying solely on their understanding of wind, thermals, and atmospheric conditions to stay above ground and travel vast distances.

Paragliding is a challenge that involves not just extended periods of flight but also strenuous mountain hikes with heavy equipment. Pilots must often ascend steep terrain to reach remote, high-altitude launch sites. This combination of hiking and flying pushes athletes to their physical and mental limits, as they need to conserve energy for long flights while tackling tough climbs on foot. Every decision made in the air is critical, with pilots scanning the horizon for thermals to gain altitude and adjusting their flight paths in response to constantly changing air currents. The unpredictable nature of weather adds another layer of difficulty, forcing pilots to adapt their strategies in real-time to navigate the skies safely and efficiently.

Lets review the hardest paragliding hike and fly races in the world.

PARAGLIDING

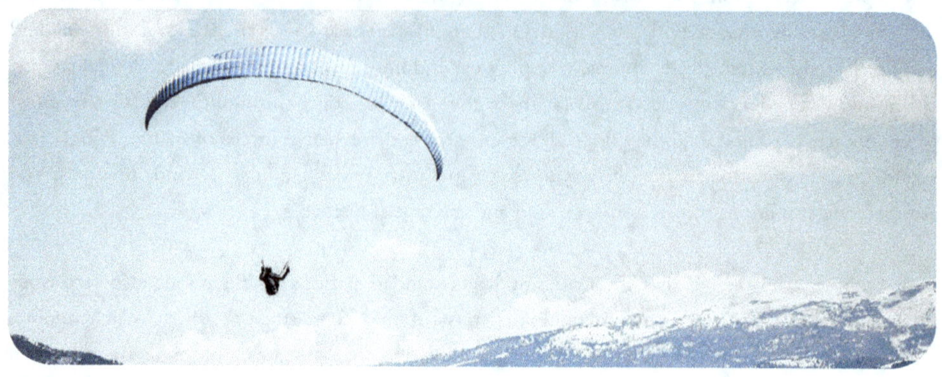

Paragliding is a thrilling aerial sport where pilots navigate their wings through a series of checkpoints or around a marked course, often over varying and challenging terrain. Unlike traditional aviation, paragliding involves launching from a hillside or elevated location and using the wind and thermals to stay airborne. In competitive racing, pilots aim to complete the course in the shortest time possible while skilfully managing their flight path to maximize speed and efficiency. Races can range from cross-country events, where pilots cover long distances from one point to another, to more technical competitions involving precision flying and strategic use of air currents. The sport combines elements of navigation, meteorology, and aerodynamics, making it a complex and dynamic challenge where skilful piloting and strategic decision-making are key to success.

Paragliding, as a sport, has its origins in the 1960s and 1970s, evolving from parachuting techniques and experimentation with wing designs. The modern form of paragliding emerged in the early 1980s when pioneers like Frenchman Pierre Lemongine developed and refined the first truly functional paraglider wings. Initially, paragliding was primarily a recreational activity, but as equipment improved and the sport gained popularity, competitive events began to take shape. The first official paragliding race took place in the late 1980s, with pilots testing their skills in various formats. Over the years, the sport has grown globally, with organized competitions and a structured racing scene established through associations such as the Paragliding World Cup (PWC) and the FAI (Fédération Aéronautique Internationale). These developments have helped standardize rules, promote safety, and enhance the competitive aspect of the sport.

The concept of long endurance races in paragliding began to take form in the 1990s, as pilots sought to push the limits of cross-country flying. One of the earliest significant events was the "Paragliding World Cup" series, which introduced a variety of long-distance races that challenged pilots to cover extensive distances while navigating through changing weather and terrain.

These early endurance races set the stage for modern cross-country paragliding, where pilots aim to fly hundreds of kilometres in a single flight, often over the course of several hours or even days. The development of accurate GPS technology and improved glider designs further fuelled these long-distance endeavours, allowing pilots to undertake increasingly ambitious routes and competitions.

Paragliding races have evolved to become more challenging due to advancements in technology, changes in competition formats, and increased pilot skill levels. Additionally, race organizers are continuously introducing new formats and challenges, such as cross-country races with multiple turn points or races that require pilots to navigate through specific waypoints under variable conditions. This evolution reflects a trend towards more demanding and diverse racing scenarios that require a combination of advanced flying skills, strategic planning, and adaptability.

The difficulty of paragliding races arises from a combination of environmental and technical factors. Environmentally, pilots must contend with fluctuating weather conditions, such as wind, turbulence, and thermal activity, which can significantly impact their flight performance and navigation. Technically, the need to manage and optimize flight dynamics, such as lift and descent rates, requires precise control and decision-making to maintain an efficient trajectory and avoid potential hazards. Additionally, once they land, there is usually a physical requirement of hiking for an extended period to reach the next flight zone. It's for this reason I believe paragliding deserves a place in the book of the worlds toughest endurance races. Let's see what events there are.

ICARUS TROPHY

- **Location**.. United States
- **Time of year**............................... September
- **Approximate distance**................. 1600km (1000 miles)
- **Average time to finish**................ 7 – 14 days
- **Average number of entries**.......... 20 – 30 participants
- **Average cost to enter**.................. $3000 – $5000
- **Year it started**............................ 2015
- **Support offered**........................... Unsupported

The Icarus Trophy is the world's longest and most challenging paramotor race, known as the ultimate test of skill, endurance, and adventure. First held in 2015, the race was conceived to push the limits of what is possible in paramotoring—a form of powered paragliding. The Icarus Trophy takes pilots on a journey over vast and varied landscapes, requiring them to navigate, plan, and fly long distances with minimal support. Unlike traditional races, the Icarus Trophy is as much about the journey as it is about the competition, with pilots often flying through remote and stunningly beautiful areas, encountering both physical and mental challenges along the way. The race has quickly gained a reputation as a must-do event for adventurous paramotor pilots, attracting participants from around the world who are eager to test their limits.

The course is not predefined, instead, pilots are given start and end points, with waypoints in between that they must reach. This means pilots must use their navigation skills to chart the best route, taking into account weather conditions, fuel availability, and terrain. Pilots must be self-sufficient, carrying all necessary equipment, fuel, and supplies. Weather conditions can vary dramatically, with pilots facing everything from calm, clear skies to strong winds, rain, and turbulence.

Entry into the Icarus Trophy is open to experienced paramotor pilots who are comfortable with long-distance flying and self-navigation. Pilots are required to carry essential gear, including GPS devices, communication equipment, and emergency supplies, and must be capable of handling any mechanical issues or emergencies that arise during the race.

You can find further details about Icarus Trophy on their official website: https://icarustrophy.com/

RED BULL X-ALPS

- **Location**.............................. Various countries
- **Time of year**.............................. June
- **Approximate distance**.................. 1000km (621 miles)
- **Average time to finish**.................. 10 – 12 days
- **Average number of entries**.......... 30 – 35 participants
- **Average cost to enter**................... Invitation only
- **Year it started**............................ 2003
- **Support offered**........................... Supported

The Red Bull X-Alps is renowned as one of the world's toughest adventure races, combining paragliding and hiking across the Alps. Since its first event in 2003, it has been held biennially and has gained a reputation for endurance and complexity. The race was created by Hannes Arch as a unique challenge to test some of the best paragliders and adventure racers in the world in an epic traverse of one of Europe's most spectacular mountain ranges.

The Red Bull X-Alps demands athletes navigate their way across the Alps, from Salzburg to Monaco, by foot or paraglider only. The route involves multiple turn points in several countries, which often includes flying over or hiking across some of the highest mountains in Europe. The strategic planning of choosing when to fly and when to hike, based on weather conditions and physical readiness, adds a significant mental challenge to the race. The unpredictable alpine weather, requiring real time decision making and adjustments, makes the race not just a physical, but a highly strategic one.

Entry to the Red Bull X-Alps is highly competitive and by invitation only. Candidates must apply by submitting detailed applications showcasing their paragliding experience, endurance racing credentials, and physical fitness levels. The selection committee, comprising experts and previous competitors, evaluates applicants based on their adventure racing and paragliding skills, past competition results, and ability to manage long-duration endurance events. Prospective athletes typically need a strong background in both cross-country paragliding and alpine endurance sports to be considered.

You can find information about the Red Bull X-Alps on their official website: https://www.redbullxalps.com/

X-PYR

- **Location**..................................... Spain
- **Time of year**............................... July
- **Approximate distance**................. 600km (373 miles)
- **Average time to finish**................ 8 – 12 days
- **Average number of entries**.......... 30 – 35 participants
- **Average cost to enter**................... $500 – $800
- **Year it started**............................. 2012
- **Support offered**........................... Semi-supported

The X-Pyr is one of the most demanding hike-and-fly paragliding races in the world, first held in 2012. The race traverses the entire length of the Pyrenees Mountains, from the Atlantic coast in the west to the Mediterranean Sea in the east. Inspired by the famous Red Bull X-Alps, the X-Pyr challenges competitors to navigate the rugged and beautiful terrain of the Pyrenees using only their paragliders and their feet. The race has quickly gained a reputation for its difficulty and the spectacular scenery it offers, attracting elite paragliders and adventurers from around the globe.

The X-Pyr course goes across the Pyrenees, from Hondarribia on the Bay of Biscay to El Port de la Selva on the Mediterranean Sea. The race is divided into several checkpoints that teams must reach, with the route between these points being determined by the pilots based on weather conditions and terrain. Competitors must balance the demands of flying in often turbulent mountain conditions with the physical exertion of hiking when flying is not possible. The Pyrenees present a range of challenges, including high-altitude passes, rapidly changing weather, strong valley winds, and the physical demands of hiking with paragliding gear. The race requires a high level of technical paragliding skill, physical endurance, and strategic decision-making.

Entry into the X-Pyr is highly competitive, with a limited number of spots available. Prospective participants must demonstrate significant experience in both paragliding and mountain navigation. The application process includes submitting a detailed resume of the pilot's experience, particularly in long-distance, hike-and-fly paragliding competitions, and mountain flying.

You can find further details about X-Pyr on their official website:
https://x-pyr.com/

VERCOFLY

- **Location**... Switzerland
- **Time of year**...................................... August
- **Approximate distance**.................. 300km (186 miles)
- **Average time to finish**.................. 3 – 6 days
- **Average number of entries**.......... 30 – 50 participants
- **Average cost to enter**................... $200 – $400
- **Year it started**............................. 2011
- **Support offered**........................... Semi-supported

Vercofly is a renowned hike-and-fly paragliding race held in the stunning Valais region of Switzerland. First organized in 2011, the race quickly gained popularity among paragliding enthusiasts for its challenging course that combines the beauty of the Swiss Alps with the demanding nature of hike-and-fly competitions. Vercofly offers a unique format where pilots must navigate through various checkpoints scattered across the Valais region, using only their paragliders and their feet. The race embodies the spirit of adventure, testing not only the pilots' flying skills but also their physical endurance and strategic planning. Over the years, Vercofly has attracted a dedicated following, making it one of the key events in the European hike-and-fly calendar.

The course starts and finishes in Vercorin, a picturesque village in the Valais region, with pilots required to reach a series of checkpoints located at strategic points across the mountains. The course is demanding due to the combination of long flights over rugged alpine terrain and strenuous hikes to reach takeoff points or cross valleys when flying conditions are unfavourable. Pilots must contend with rapidly changing weather, strong valley winds, and the technical challenges of flying in high-altitude mountain environments. The physical demands are equally intense, as participants often hike with heavy paragliding equipment, navigating steep ascents and descents.

Entry into Vercofly is open to experienced paragliders who have a proven track record in hike-and-fly or cross-country paragliding competitions. Applicants are typically required to demonstrate their experience through a detailed resume, including previous race results, long-distance flights, and experience in mountainous terrain.

You can find further details about Vercofly on their official website:
https://www.vercofly.ch/

TRANSDROMOISE

- **Location**.. France
- **Time of year**................................... May
- **Approximate distance**.................. 200km (124 miles)
- **Average time to finish**................. 2 – 3 days
- **Average number of entries**........... 50 participants
- **Average cost to enter**................... $150 – $300
- **Year it started**............................. 2015
- **Support offered**........................... Semi-supported

Transdromoise is a hike-and-fly paragliding race held in the picturesque Drôme region of France. First launched in 2015, this race has quickly become a popular event among the European paragliding community for its combination of challenging terrain, beautiful landscapes, and the unique format that requires participants to use both their flying and hiking skills to navigate the course. The event is typically organized in late spring, when the weather conditions in the Drôme are ideal for both paragliding and long-distance trekking.

The race is structured around multiple checkpoints that participants must reach, with the route between these points being largely up to the competitors. This flexibility allows pilots to choose between flying and hiking based on weather conditions and terrain. The course is challenging due to the combination of technical flying in mountainous terrain and the physical demands of hiking with paragliding equipment. Participants must navigate steep ascents and descents, and often contend with rapidly changing weather conditions, including strong valley winds and thermals. The difficulty is further enhanced by the need to make strategic decisions about when to fly and when to hike, balancing the risks and rewards of each option.

While there are no formal qualifying requirements, participants are expected to have significant experience in mountain flying and long-distance trekking.

You can find details about Transdromoise on their official website:
https://www.transdromoise.fr/

BORNES TO FLY

- **Location**.................................... France
- **Time of year**.............................. May
- **Approximate distance**................. 130km (81 miles)
- **Average time to finish**................. 2 – 3 days
- **Average number of entries**.......... 50 – 60 participants
- **Average cost to enter**.................. $150 – $200
- **Year it started**............................ 2013
- **Support offered**.......................... Semi-supported

Bornes to Fly is a hike-and-fly paragliding race that takes place in the picturesque Bornes Massif region of Haute-Savoie, France. First held in 2013, the race has quickly become a favourite among the European hike-and-fly community for its challenging terrain and breathtaking scenery. The race has steadily grown in popularity, with more participants each year eager to take on the unique challenges that the Bornes Massif has to offer.

The Bornes to Fly course covers approximately 130km through the varied terrain of the Bornes Massif. The race begins and ends in the town of Talloires, located on the shores of Lake Annecy, which provides a stunning backdrop for the competition. The course is designed to test the full range of a pilot's abilities, combining long flights over mountainous terrain with challenging hikes to reach the best takeoff points. Participants must navigate through multiple checkpoints scattered across the region, often requiring steep climbs and descents, navigating through forests, and dealing with the unpredictable alpine weather. Strong valley winds, thermals, and rapidly changing weather conditions can turn what seems like a straightforward flight into a complex challenge, requiring both technical flying skills and physical endurance.

Entry into Bornes to Fly is open to experienced paragliders who are comfortable with the demands of long-distance hike-and-fly competitions. The entry fee ranges from EUR 150 to 250, depending on the level of support and services provided during the race. All participants are required to carry essential safety equipment, including a GPS tracker, radio, and emergency supplies, ensuring they are prepared for the rigors of the race.

You can find further details about Bornes To Fly on their official website: https://www.bornestofly.fr/

X-SCOTIA HIKE AND FLY

- **Location**.. Scotland
- **Time of year**............................... June
- **Approximate distance**................. 100km (60 miles)
- **Average time to finish**................. 2 days
- **Average number of entries**.......... 50 participants
- **Average cost to enter**................... $100 – $200
- **Year it started**.............................. 2018
- **Support offered**............................ Semi-supported

The X-Scotia Hike and Fly is a unique adventure race that takes place in the beautiful landscapes of the Scottish Highlands. First organized in 2018, the race has quickly gained popularity among paragliding enthusiasts who are drawn to the challenge of combining hiking with flying across Scotland's iconic mountains and glens. Inspired by events such as the Red Bull X-Alps, the X-Scotia is part of the growing "hike-and-fly" discipline, which requires participants to navigate long distances by alternating between hiking on foot and flying by paraglider. The race is designed to test the endurance, navigation skills, and flying expertise of the participants as they traverse some of Scotland's most remote terrain.

The course changes each year but typically covers between 50 and 100km, with competitors tasked with reaching various checkpoints scattered throughout the Scottish Highlands. The weather in the Scottish Highlands is notoriously changeable, and pilots must be highly skilled at assessing when it's safe to launch and fly. The hike portions can be tough, often requiring competitors to climb steep mountains with their paragliding gear on their backs. The unpredictable weather, combined with the remote and mountainous terrain, makes X-Scotia one of the toughest hike-and-fly events, requiring not only excellent paragliding skills but also strong physical fitness and a deep knowledge of navigation and mountain safety.

There are no formal qualification requirements, but participants must be competent in both paragliding and mountain navigation, and they should be prepared for the challenges of flying in unpredictable Scottish weather.

You can find further details about X-Scotia on their official website: https://x-scotia.co.uk/

CHAPTER 3 – SNOW SPORTS

In Chapter 3, we examine some of the world's toughest snow sports, where athletes are pushed to their limits in some of the harshest environments on Earth. Competing in freezing temperatures, unpredictable weather, and at high altitudes in mountainous terrain demands a unique combination of strength, stamina, and mental resilience. These athletes must not only contend with the natural elements but also manage their own physical endurance as they tackle difficult and often dangerous conditions.

This chapter explores sports like ski mountaineering, cross-country skiing, and ice skating, each of which challenges athletes to balance intense physical exertion with technical skill. Ski mountaineering combines the endurance of long uphill climbs with the need for rapid, steep descents, often in environments where the terrain is both treacherous and unpredictable. Cross-country skiing, on the other hand, requires athletes to maintain a steady pace over long distances, battling through snow and wind while pushing their bodies to exhaustion. Ice skating, while different, similarly demands a blend of power and control as skaters navigate slippery surfaces with speed and precision.

 Together, these snow sports demonstrate the extraordinary physical and mental fortitude required to compete in winter's most extreme conditions. Whether ascending snowy peaks, racing across endless trails, or performing on ice, athletes are continuously forced to adapt to the unique challenges of their environment. These sports require a delicate balance of power, endurance, and technical finesse, showcasing the remarkable abilities of those who participate.

In each of these disciplines, athletes are pushed beyond what most people would consider humanly possible. Whether it's the explosive energy needed to scale a mountain on skis, the relentless pace of a cross-country marathon, or the precision required for ice skating, these winter sports represent the pinnacle of endurance in cold, unforgiving conditions. Through this exploration, we gain a greater appreciation for the athletes who thrive in such extreme environments, continually pushing the boundaries of what can be achieved in the most hostile climates on the planet. Let's look into what the toughest races in the world on snow are.

ICE SKATING

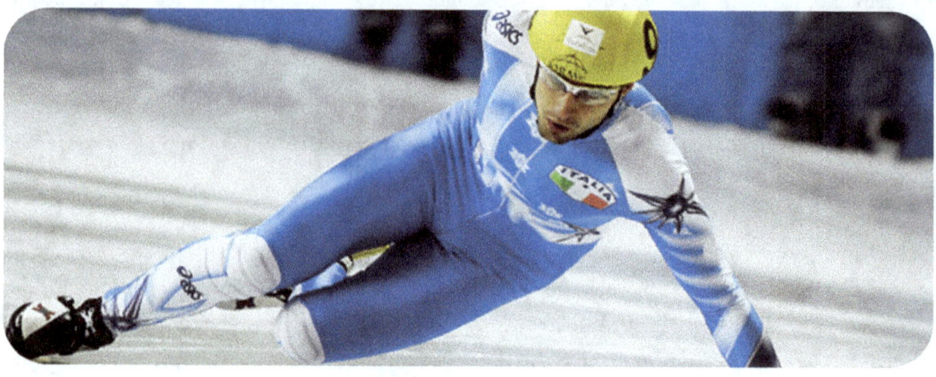

Ice skating, particularly in the context of long-distance endurance races, is a sport which combines sustained speed and endurance over extended distances on ice. Unlike shorter sprint events that focus on explosive speed and technique, long-distance ice-skating races require athletes to maintain their performance over hours or even days. These races are typically held on natural ice surfaces, such as frozen lakes and rivers, which means lots of variability in the conditions. These races can span from a few kilometres to over 200km, with events like the Elfstedentocht in the Netherlands being the iconic example. The strategic aspect of pacing, combined with the need for technical skill to handle a range of ice surfaces and environmental factors, makes long-distance ice skating racing a test of endurance and skill.

The earliest evidence of ice skating dates to 3000 BC in Scandinavia, where people used sharpened bones strapped to their feet to glide over frozen lakes and rivers allowing humans to travel more efficiently. By the 17th century, the Dutch made significant advancements by introducing metal blades, which enabled more faster skating. Ice skating quickly evolved into a popular sport and leisure activity, with formal competitions beginning to take shape in the 19th century. Organized events and standardized rules marked the transition of ice skating from a practical activity to a competitive sport, laying the groundwork for modern figure skating and speed skating.

Long endurance ice skating races first gained prominence in the late 19th century, particularly in the Netherlands, where the sport has historical roots. These early races were held on natural ice and could span considerable distances, often ranging from 50 to over 200km. One of the most notable early endurance races is the Elfstedentocht, which involves skating through eleven cities in Friesland and covering approximately 200km. This race, first held in 1909, quickly became a celebrated event.

Endurance ice skating races have evolved significantly over the years, becoming increasingly demanding due to advancements in technology, training, and course design. Modern races often feature longer distances and more complex routes, which may include variations in ice quality and challenging weather conditions. Advances in equipment, such as specialized blades designed for optimal glide and energy efficiency, have pushed the limits of what distances and speeds skaters can achieve. Additionally, improved training methods and a deeper understanding of sports science have raised the level of competition, with athletes now required to perform at peak levels over extended periods. The evolution of these races reflects a trend toward greater endurance challenges.

The difficulty of endurance ice skating races stems from a combination of factors. Physically, skaters must maintain endurance over long distances, often on ice that can vary in quality from smooth to rough. Environmental challenges include the potential weather conditions skaters may encounter such as strong winds and freezing temperatures. Through the combination of these factors I believe the following races are the toughest ice skating races in the world. Let's take a look.

WEISSENSEE

- Location...................................... Austria
- Time of year............................... February
- Approximate distance................. 200km (124 miles)
- Average time to finish................. 7 – 10 hours
- Average number of entries.......... 3000 – 4000 participants
- Average cost to enter................... $50 – $150
- Year it started............................. 1989
- Support offered........................... Supported

The Weissensee Ice Skating Race is one of the most prestigious and challenging natural ice-skating events in the world, held annually on the frozen Weissensee in Carinthia, Austria. Established in 1989, the event was inspired by the Dutch tradition of long-distance ice-skating marathons, particularly the Elfstedentocht. Over the years, Weissensee has become known as the "Alternative Elfstedentocht" due to its popularity among Dutch skaters, many of whom flock to Austria to train and compete in the event. The race has grown significantly since its inception and now features a variety of distances, culminating in the gruelling 200km marathon. This event is celebrated not just for its competitive nature, but also for its beautiful Alpine setting, making it a bucket-list race for long-distance skaters.

The race takes place on a large, frozen lake nestled in the Austrian Alps. The course is typically set up in long loops around the lake, with skaters completing multiple laps to reach the full distance. One of the key challenges of the race is the natural ice itself, which can vary in quality depending on the weather conditions leading up to and during the event. The ice can range from smooth and fast to rough and bumpy, with potential cracks and snow-covered sections adding to the difficulty. The weather in January and February can be harsh, with temperatures often dropping well below freezing.

The race is open to skaters of all levels, with various distances available to accommodate different abilities. While there are no formal qualification requirements, participants in the longer races, especially the 200km event, are expected to have considerable experience in long-distance skating.

You can find details about Weissensee on their official website:
https://www.weissensee.com/en/

BAIKAL WILD ICE GRAND MARATHON

- **Location**...................................... Russia
- **Time of year**................................ March
- **Approximate distance**................. 200km (124 miles)
- **Average time to finish**............... 10 – 14 hours
- **Average number of entries**.......... 100 – 150 participants
- **Average cost to enter**.................. $800 – $1200
- **Year it started**............................. 2010
- **Support offered**........................... Supported

The Baikal Wild Ice Skating Grand Marathon is one of the most extraordinary and challenging ice skating events in the world, held annually on the frozen surface of Lake Baikal, the oldest and deepest freshwater lake on the planet. Launched in 2010, the event was created to celebrate the beauty of Lake Baikal in winter and to offer a unique endurance challenge to long-distance ice skaters. Over the years, the marathon has gained a reputation for being one of the toughest natural ice marathons, attracting skaters from all over the world.

The course is laid out on the vast, frozen expanse of Lake Baikal, stretching over 200km from one side of the lake to the other. The ice is typically 1.5 to 2 meters thick, but its surface can vary widely, ranging from perfectly smooth, clear ice to rough, snow-covered sections that are challenging to navigate. The race takes place in March, when temperatures can still be extremely cold, often ranging from -15°C to -25°C (5°F to -13°F), with the wind adding to the difficulty by creating additional resistance and lowering the effective temperature. The vastness of the lake means that skaters are often isolated, with little to no visual markers except the distant shorelines.

While there are no formal qualification times required to enter the race, participants are expected to have substantial experience in long-distance ice skating and be in excellent physical condition. The marathon demands not only skating proficiency but also the ability to endure long hours in harsh weather. Participants must bring appropriate gear, including specialized skates designed for long-distance and rough ice, and equipment to carry necessary supplies during the race.

You can find details about the Baikal Ice Marathon on their official website:
https://baikalcomplex.com/skatemarathon

FINLAND ICE MARATHON

- **Location**...................................... Finland
- **Time of year**............................... February
- **Approximate distance**................. 200km (124 miles)
- **Average time to finish**................ 7 – 8 hours
- **Average number of entries**.......... 300 – 500 participants
- **Average cost to enter**................... $50 – $100
- **Year it started**............................. 1984
- **Support offered**........................... Supported

The Finland Ice Marathon is a historic ice skating race held annually in Kuopio, Finland. Established in 1984, it is one of the oldest and most prestigious ice marathon events in the world. The race takes place on the natural ice of Lake Kallavesi, offering participants the unique experience of skating through the picturesque Finnish winter landscape. Over the years, the event has grown to include various race distances, catering to both elite skaters and recreational participants. The Finland Ice Marathon has become a key event in the Finnish winter sports calendar, attracting skaters from across Europe and beyond, all eager to test their endurance on the ice.

The course is laid out on the frozen surface of Lake Kallavesi, creating a challenging experience for participants. The main event is the 200km race, which involves multiple laps around the lake. The difficulty of the race lies in the unpredictable conditions of natural ice. Depending on the weather leading up to the event, the ice can be smooth and fast, or it can be rough, cracked, and difficult to skate on. Skaters must also contend with the cold, often facing temperatures well below freezing, and the wind, which can be strong and relentless across the open lake.

The Finland Ice Marathon is open to skaters of all levels, with various distances available to suit different abilities. While there are no strict entry requirements, participants in the longer races, especially the 200km marathon, are expected to have significant experience in long-distance skating or endurance sports. The organizers provide comprehensive support, including medical assistance and rest areas, but skaters must be self-sufficient and prepared for the rigors of the race.

You can find details about the Finland Ice Marathon on their official website:

https://www.finlandicemarathon.com/

SKATE THE LAKE

- **Location**............................ Canada
- **Time of year**.............................. January
- **Approximate distance**................. 75km (46.6 miles)
- **Average time to finish**................. 3 – 6 hours
- **Average number of entries**.......... 300 – 500 participants
- **Average cost to enter**.................. $40 – $100
- **Year it started**............................ 2004
- **Support offered**.......................... Supported

Skate the Lake is an annual long-distance ice skating event held in Portland, Ontario, on the frozen Big Rideau Lake. The event, first established in 2004, has grown in popularity and is now a cornerstone of the Canadian winter sports calendar. Conceived to celebrate the tradition of long-distance skating, particularly in the Dutch style of marathons on natural ice, Skate the Lake draws skaters from across North America and even Europe. Over the years, the event has expanded to include various race distances, accommodating everyone from casual skaters to elite competitors.

The course for Skate the Lake is laid out on Big Rideau Lake, where the natural ice can vary significantly in quality and thickness depending on weather conditions. The course is typically a large loop, with skaters completing multiple laps to achieve the full race distance. One of the key challenges of this race is the unpredictable nature of the ice. Even with careful preparation, the surface can be uneven, cracked, or affected by snowdrifts, making it difficult to maintain speed and balance. Additionally, the race is held in late January, when temperatures in this region of Canada can plunge well below freezing, with wind chills that can sap energy and test the endurance of even the most seasoned skaters.

Skate the Lake is open to skaters of all levels, from beginners to elite athletes. There are no strict entry requirements in terms of qualification times or previous race experience. However, given the extreme cold and the demanding nature of the course, participants are strongly encouraged to have some experience with long-distance skating or endurance sports.

You can find details about Skate the Lake on their official website: https://www.portlandoutdoors.com/

CROSS COUNTRY SKIING

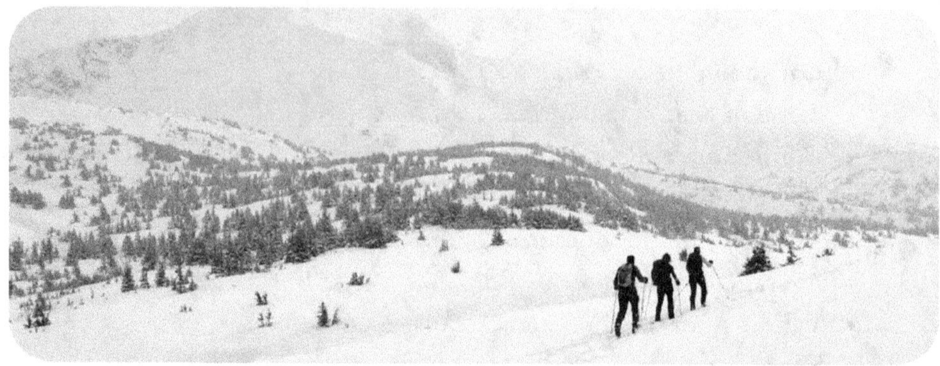

Cross-country ski racing is a winter sport where athletes navigate long distances across varied snow-covered terrain using skis and poles. Unlike alpine skiing, which focuses on downhill speed and turns, cross-country skiing emphasizes endurance, technique, and efficiency on flat or rolling terrain. Races can range from short sprints to marathon-length events, challenging skiers to balance speed, stamina, and technique. The sport includes different disciplines such as freestyle (skating technique) and classical (traditional diagonal stride), each requiring distinct skills and training. The combination of aerobic endurance, strength, and technical proficiency makes cross-country skiing racing a comprehensive test of athleticism.

Cross-country skiing has roots in ancient Scandinavia, where it was originally developed as a means of transportation across snowy landscapes. Evidence suggests that the practice dates back over 4,000 years, with early skis made from wood or bone. It wasn't until the 19th century that cross-country skiing evolved into a competitive sport, with formal races and events beginning to take shape in Norway, a country renowned for its skiing tradition. The sport gained international recognition with the founding of the International Ski Federation (FIS) in 1924, which began organizing world championships and setting standardized rules. Cross-country skiing was featured in the first Winter Olympics in 1924, further cementing its status as a global competitive sport. Since then, it has grown in popularity, with advancements in equipment and technique continually shaping its development.

The first long endurance cross-country skiing races began to take form in the early 20th century, reflecting the sport's deep-rooted traditions and the increasing interest in competitive events. One of the earliest and most significant long-distance races is the Vasaloppet, held in Sweden since 1922.

This iconic race, named in honor of the historical Swedish figure Gustav Vasa, covers 90km and traverses challenging terrain from Sälen to Mora. Similarly, the Birkebeiner Race in Norway, which originated in 1932, offers a 54km course and pays homage to historical events. These early races set the stage for the evolution of endurance events, establishing benchmarks for distance and difficulty.

Cross-country skiing races have evolved significantly, with modern events featuring increased distances, more demanding courses, and advanced technology. Contemporary races often include a variety of challenging terrains, such as steep ascents, technical descents, and varied snow conditions, which test skiers' skill. Technological advancements in equipment, including lighter and more efficient skis, poles, and clothing, have pushed performance boundaries, making races more competitive.

The difficulty of cross-country skiing races stems from a combination of physical, environmental, and technical challenges. Physically, the races demand exceptional aerobic endurance and strength, as skiers must maintain a high level of exertion over long distances and varying terrain. Environmental factors, such as changing snow conditions, weather extremes and altitude. Technical skills are crucial for handling diverse terrain, including uphill climbs, downhill descents, and variable snow conditions. The mental aspect also plays a significant role, as skiers must stay focused and motivated despite fatigue and discomfort. The interplay of these factors makes cross-country skiing races a rigorous test of overall fitness, skill, and mental resilience.

NORDENSKIÖLDSLOPPET

- **Location**...................................... Sweden
- **Time of year**............................... March
- **Approximate distance**................. 220km (137 miles)
- **Average time to finish**................. 12 – 30 hours
- **Average number of entries**.......... 400 – 500 participants
- **Average cost to enter**................... $250 – $350
- **Year it started**............................ 1884
- **Support offered**.......................... Supported

The Nordenskiöldsloppet is the world's longest cross-country ski race, held annually in the stunning wilderness of Swedish Lapland. First organized in 1884 by polar explorer Adolf Erik Nordenskiöld, the race was designed to be an extreme test of endurance, inspired by a 460km ski expedition he led in Greenland. After lying dormant for over a century, the race was revived in 2016. Today, the Nordenskiöldsloppet is recognized as one of the most challenging ski races globally, attracting elite skiers and amateurs.

The Nordenskiöldsloppet spans an incredible 220km through the snowy wilderness of Swedish Lapland, starting and finishing in Jokkmokk, a small town just north of the Arctic Circle. The course takes skiers across frozen lakes, through dense forests, and over rolling hills, all while navigating the challenges of deep snow, sub-zero temperatures, and the possibility of strong winds and blizzards.

While there are no specific qualifying requirements, participants are strongly encouraged to have completed long-distance ski races and to be in excellent physical condition. Safety is a top priority, with medical teams and safety personnel stationed at various points along the route, as well as snowmobiles and other vehicles available for emergency evacuations if necessary.

You can find details about the Nordenskiöldsloppet on their official website: https://www.nordenskioldsloppet.com/

ARCTIC CIRCLE SKI RACE

- **Location**.. Greenland
- **Time of year**.................................. April
- **Approximate distance**.................. 160km (100 miles)
- **Average time to finish**................. 3 days (6 – 12hr per day)
- **Average number of entries**.......... 50 – 100 participants
- **Average cost to enter**................... $600 – $1000
- **Year it started**............................. 1998
- **Support offered**........................... Supported

The Arctic Circle Ski Race is one of the most remote cross-country ski races in the world, held annually in the vast wilderness of Greenland. Established in 1998, the race was designed to attract adventurous skiers who are eager to test their endurance in one of the planet's most extreme environments. The event takes place near the town of Sisimiut, located just north of the Arctic Circle, and participants are required to ski 160km over the course of three days.

The course winds through remote Arctic landscapes, including frozen fjords, towering mountains, and vast, snow-covered tundra. Participants must navigate the unpredictable Arctic weather, which can range from clear skies and bright sunshine to blizzards, high winds, and temperatures that can plummet far below freezing. The race is divided into three stages, with each stage covering between 50 to 60km. The isolation of the course adds another layer of difficulty, participants are often far from any settlements, relying solely on the support provided at checkpoints.

Entry into the race is open to experienced cross-country skiers who are prepared to handle the extreme conditions and physical demands of the event. While there are no formal qualification requirements, participants are strongly encouraged to have experience in long-distance skiing and to be in excellent physical condition.

You can find details about the Arctic Circle Ski race on their official website: https://acr.gl/

CANADIAN SKI MARATHON

- **Location**..................................... Canada
- **Time of year**............................... February
- **Approximate distance**.................. 160km (99 miles)
- **Average time to finish**.................. 2 days (6 – 10 hours per day)
- **Average number of entries**.......... 2000 – 3000 participants
- **Average cost to enter**................... $200 – $350
- **Year it started**............................. 1967
- **Support offered**........................... Supported

The Canadian Ski Marathon (CSM) is the longest and oldest Nordic ski tour in North America, offering a non-competitive yet challenging adventure through the countryside of Quebec. First held in 1967 as part of Canada's centennial celebrations, the CSM has become an annual event, attracting skiers from across Canada and around the world. The marathon is unique in its format, being a two-day tour that covers 160km of pisted trails, divided into 10 sections. Unlike a typical race, the CSM is a personal challenge, with participants striving to complete as many sections as they can, at their own pace, within the allotted time each day.

The course stretches 160km from Lachute to Gatineau, traversing the rolling hills, dense forests, and open fields of Quebec's Laurentian region. It's divided into 10 sections, with participants skiing five sections each day, covering roughly 80km per day. While the terrain is generally rolling, it includes a mix of challenging climbs and descents.

Entry into the Canadian Ski Marathon is open to skiers of all levels, from seasoned Nordic skiers to beginners looking for a unique challenge. There are no formal qualification requirements, but participants should be in good physical condition and prepared for long days on the trails. The event offers various participation categories, including the full marathon, half marathon, and shorter distances for those looking for a less demanding experience. For those seeking the ultimate challenge, the CSM includes the prestigious "Coureur des Bois" categories, where skiers carry all their gear and, in the gold category, camp overnight on the trail.

You can find details about the Canadian Ski Marathon on their official website: https://skimarathon.ca/

VASALOPPET

- **Location**.. Sweden
- **Time of year**.................................. March
- **Approximate distance**.................. 90km (56 miles)
- **Average time to finish**.................. 4 – 10 hours
- **Average number of entries**.......... 15,000 – 16,000
- **Average cost to enter**.................... $170 – $230
- **Year it started**.............................. 1922
- **Support offered**............................ Supported

The Vasaloppet is the oldest cross-country ski races in the world. Held annually in Sweden, the race covers 90km from Sälen to Mora, following a historic route inspired by King Gustav Vasa's legendary journey in 1521. It is the largest cross-country ski race in the world as well and serves as the pinnacle of the annual "Vasaloppet Week," which includes a series of races for different levels and disciplines. The Vasaloppet is also part of the Worldloppet series, making it a key event in the international ski marathon calendar. The race is a celebration of Swedish history and culture, with its roots deeply embedded in the country's national identity.

The course goes through the snow-covered forests and fields of Dalarna, from Sälen in the west to Mora in the east. The terrain is varied, featuring long flat sections, gentle climbs, and a few steeper ascents, particularly in the early stages of the race. The most famous climb is the initial 3-kilometer uphill stretch from the start, which sets the tone for the endurance required throughout the race. The sheer number of participants also adds to the difficulty, especially at the start, where skiers must jostle for position.

Entry into the Vasaloppet is open to skiers of all levels, from elite athletes to recreational participants, although spots are highly sought after and often sell out quickly. Participants receive extensive support, including food and hydration stations along the course, waxing services, and medical teams stationed at various points. The race is well-organized, with timing chips to track progress and a festive atmosphere in both Sälen and Mora, where spectators cheer on the skiers.

You can find details about Vasaloppet on their official website:
https://www.vasaloppet.se/en/

LA TRANSJURASSIENNE

- **Location**.. France
- **Time of year**................................. February
- **Approximate distance**................. 70km (43.5 miles)
- **Average time to finish**................ 3 – 6 hours
- **Average number of entries**.......... 4000 – 5000 participants
- **Average cost to enter**.................. $70 – $100
- **Year it started**............................. 1979
- **Support offered**........................... Supported

La Transjurassienne is one of the most iconic cross-country ski races in France and is a key event in the international ski marathon circuit. First held in 1979, the race takes place in the Jura Mountains, a stunning region known for its rolling hills, dense forests, and picturesque villages. As part of the Worldloppet series, La Transjurassienne attracts both elite athletes and recreational skiers from around the world. Over the years, the race has grown in popularity and now includes multiple distances and styles, making it accessible to a wide range of participants.

The main event is a 70km race that typically starts in Lamoura and finishes in Mouthe, traversing the varied terrain of the Jura Mountains. The course is known for its challenging profile, featuring a series of long climbs, technical descents, and flat sections where skiers must maintain a high pace. The most demanding part of the course is often the ascent to the highest point at La Combe du Lac. Additionally, the Jura Mountains are known for their unpredictable weather, with skiers potentially facing anything from deep snow and cold temperatures to icy conditions and strong winds.

Entry into La Transjurassienne is open to skiers of all levels, from elite competitors to recreational participants. The race is well-organized, with timing chips provided to track progress and a festive atmosphere at the finish line in Mouthe, where skiers are greeted with cheers from spectators.

You can find details about the La Transjurassienne race on their official website: https://www.latransju.com/en

MARCIALONGA

- **Location**... Italy
- **Time of year**............................... January
- **Approximate distance**................. 70km (43.5 miles)
- **Average time to finish**................. 3 – 6 hours
- **Average number of entries**.......... 7000 – 8000 participants
- **Average cost to enter**................... $100 – $150
- **Year it started**............................. 1971
- **Support offered**........................... Supported

The Marcialonga is one of the most famous and beloved cross-country ski races in Italy and a key event in the international ski marathon calendar. The race takes place in the picturesque valleys of Fiemme and Fassa in the Trentino region. The Marcialonga has become a symbol of Italian winter sports, attracting thousands of skiers from around the world, including elite athletes.

The Marcialonga course starts in the town of Moena and finishes in Cavalese. The route takes skiers through the stunning Val di Fassa and Val di Fiemme, passing through several charming mountain villages and offering breathtaking views of the Dolomite mountains. One of the most demanding parts of the course is the final climb, known as the "Cascata," a steep ascent of approximately 2km before the finish in Cavalese. This final stretch tests the endurance and strength of even the most experienced skiers, coming after nearly 68km of skiing.

Entry is open to skiers of all levels, but spots are highly sought after, and the race often sells out quickly. The race provides extensive support for participants, including food and hydration stations, waxing services, and medical teams along the course. Timing chips are used to track participants' progress, and the event concludes with a festive atmosphere in Cavalese, where skiers are welcomed with warm Italian hospitality.

You can find details about the Marcialonga race on their official website: https://www.marcialonga.it

FINLANDIA-HIIHTO

- **Location**.. Finland
- **Time of year**................................... February
- **Approximate distance**.................. 70km (43.5 miles)
- **Average time to finish**.................. 3 – 6 hours
- **Average number of entries**........... 4000 – 5000 participants
- **Average cost to enter**.................... $70 – $100
- **Year it started**.............................. 1974
- **Support offered**............................ Supported

The Finlandia-Hiihto is one of Finland's premier cross-country ski events and an essential part of the international ski marathon circuit. First organized in 1974, this race is a celebration of Finland's rich skiing tradition and is held annually in Lahti, a city renowned for its winter sports. The race is known for its well-organized events, diverse participation distance options, and the beautiful, snowy landscapes of the Lahti region.

The Finlandia-Hiihto's main course is a 70km route that winds through the forests and rolling terrain around Lahti. The course is challenging due to its length and the varying topography, which includes long stretches of flat terrain, gradual climbs, and fast descents. The race takes place in late February when the snow conditions can vary, with temperatures often below freezing. The race is known for its well-maintained tracks, but the sheer number of participants can create crowded conditions, especially in the early stages of the race.

Entry into the Finlandia-Hiihto is open to skiers of all levels, from seasoned professionals to enthusiastic amateurs. The event concludes with post-race amenities in Lahti, where skiers can enjoy a warm welcome and celebrate their achievements.

You can find details about the Finlandia-Hiihto on their official website:
https://www.finlandiahiihto.fi/

TARTU SKI MARATHON

- **Location**.. Estonia
- **Time of year**................................. February
- **Approximate distance**.................. 63km (39 miles)
- **Average time to finish**................. 3 – 5 hours
- **Average number of entries**........... 5000 – 6000 participants
- **Average cost to enter**.................... $50 – $100
- **Year it started**............................. 1960
- **Support offered**........................... Supported

The Tartu Ski Marathon is one of the oldest cross-country ski races in Eastern Europe, held annually in the forests of southern Estonia. Established in 1960, the event has become a major fixture in the Worldloppet series, which includes the most renowned ski marathons worldwide. The Tartu Ski Marathon is the largest skiing event in the Baltics, drawing thousands of participants from across Europe and beyond.

The race starts in the village of Otepää, known as Estonia's winter capital, and finishes in Elva, taking skiers through a scenic and varied landscape. The course is challenging due to its length and the undulating terrain, which includes a mix of steady climbs, fast descents, and flat sections where skiers must maintain a strong pace. The varying snow conditions typical of the region can add to the difficulty, with participants needing to adapt to anything from fresh powder to icy tracks.

Entry into the Tartu Ski Marathon is open to skiers of all levels, from elite athletes to recreational enthusiasts. There are no specific qualification requirements, making the race accessible to everyone. The event concludes with a festive atmosphere at the finish line in Elva, where skiers are welcomed with traditional Estonian hospitality and post-race celebrations.

You can find details about the Tartu Ski Marathon on their official website: https://tartumaraton.ee/en/tartu-maraton-2024

AMERICAN BIRKENBEINER

- **Location**... Wisconsin (USA)
- **Time of year**.............................. February
- **Approximate distance**................ 55km (34 miles)
- **Average time to finish**............... 2 – 5 hours
- **Average number of entries**.......... 10,000 – 13,000 participants
- **Average cost to enter**.................. $135 – $200
- **Year it started**............................. 1973
- **Support offered**........................... Supported

The American Birkebeiner, often referred to as the "Birkie," is the largest cross-country ski race in North America. The race was inspired by the Norwegian Birkebeinerrennet, a historic event that honours the 1206 rescue of the infant prince Haakon Haakonsson. The American Birkebeiner is held annually in Hayward, Wisconsin, and has grown to become a major event in the global ski marathon calendar, attracting thousands of skiers from around the world. The Birkie has a week of events leading up to the main race, including shorter races, youth events, and a vibrant festival atmosphere.

The American Birkebeiner course is known for its challenging terrain, winding through the rolling hills and forests of northern Wisconsin. The main race is a point-to-point course that starts in Cable and finishes in Hayward, covering either 50km for the Skate race or 55km for the Classic race. The course includes a mix of long climbs, fast descents, and flat sections that require both endurance and technical skill. One of the most famous features of the course is the climb up "Powerline Hill," a long and steady ascent early in the race that tests the strength and pacing of all participants. The race also includes a crossing over Lake Hayward.

Entry into the American Birkebeiner is open to skiers of all levels, but the race is particularly popular, and spots often sell out quickly. There are no specific qualification requirements. The event culminates in a festive atmosphere in downtown Hayward, where skiers are welcomed by cheering crowds and can enjoy post-race amenities.

You can find details about the American Birkebeiner on their official website: https://www.birkie.com/

BIRKEBEINERRENNET

- **Location**............................... Norway
- **Time of year**.............................. March
- **Approximate distance**................ 54km (33.5 miles)
- **Average time to finish**................ 3 – 6 hours
- **Average number of entries**.......... 10,000 – 15,000 participants
- **Average cost to enter**................... $150 – $200
- **Year it started**............................ 1932
- **Support offered**.......................... Supported

First organized in 1932, the Birkebeinerrennet commemorates a historic event from 1206, during the Norwegian civil war, when two Birkebeiner warriors carried the infant heir to the Norwegian throne, Prince Haakon Haakonsson, over the mountains to safety. The race covers 54km from Rena to Lillehammer, and participants are required to carry a backpack weighing at least 3.5kg, symbolizing the weight of the infant prince. The Birkebeinerrennet is part of the "Birkebeiner Triple," which also includes a mountain bike race and a running race, making it a significant event in Norway's sporting calendar. It is also a part of the Worldloppet series.

The course goes through the mountainous terrain from Rena to Lillehammer. It's known for its challenging climbs, particularly the ascent to the highest point at Midtfjellet, which stands at 910 meters above sea level. The combination of steep climbs, fast descents, and varying snow conditions requires a high level of fitness, endurance, and technical skill.

Entry into the Birkebeinerrennet is open to skiers of all levels, from elite athletes to recreational participants, but the race is particularly popular and often fills up quickly. Participants receive extensive support throughout the race, including food and hydration stations, waxing services, and medical assistance. Completing the Birkebeinerrennet is considered a significant achievement, with participants joining a long tradition of endurance and that dates back over 800 years. The race is more than just a sporting event; it is a tribute to Norwegian history and the spirit of the Birkebeiner warriors.

You can find details about the Birkebeinerrennet on their official website:
https://birkebeiner.no/en/ski/birkebeinerrennet-54-km

KÖNIG LUDWIG LAUF

- **Location**.................................. Germany
- **Time of year**............................. February
- **Approximate distance**................. 50km (31 miles)
- **Average time to finish**............... 2 – 5 hours
- **Average number of entries**.......... 3500 participants
- **Average cost to enter**.................. $50 – $100
- **Year it started**........................... 1968
- **Support offered**.......................... Supported

The König Ludwig Lauf is one of Germany's most popular cross-country ski races, held annually in the picturesque Bavarian town of Oberammergau. Named after King Ludwig II of Bavaria, the race was first organized in 1968 and has since become a key event in the international ski marathon calendar. It is part of the Worldloppet series, a collection of the world's most renowned ski marathons. The race attracts both elite athletes and recreational skiers, offering them the opportunity to compete in a stunning alpine setting full of history and tradition. Over the years, the König Ludwig Lauf has grown to include multiple race distances and styles, making it accessible to skiers of all ages and skill levels.

The 50km classic style race that takes skiers through some of Bavaria's most beautiful landscapes, including the Ammergau Alps and along the banks of the River Ammer. The race attracts a large field of competitors, which can make for crowded conditions on the narrow trails, particularly in the early stages. Despite these challenges, the König Ludwig Lauf is celebrated for its well-organized and festive atmosphere, with spectators lining the course and a strong sense of camaraderie among participants.

Entry into the König Ludwig Lauf is open to skiers of all levels, from elite competitors to recreational participants. There are no specific qualification requirements. The race is well-supported, with multiple food and hydration stations along the course, as well as medical and safety teams on hand to assist. Skiers are also provided with timing chips to track their progress, and the event concludes with a celebratory atmosphere in Oberammergau, where participants can enjoy post-race festivities and traditional Bavarian hospitality.

You can find details about the König Ludwig Lauf race on their official website:
https://www.koenig-ludwig-lauf.com/

ENGADIN SKIMARATHON

- **Location**.. Switzerland
- **Time of year**................................... March
- **Approximate distance**................. 42km (26 miles)
- **Average time to finish**................. 2 – 3 hours
- **Average number of entries**.......... 14,000 – 15,000 participants
- **Average cost to enter**................... $100 – $150
- **Year it started**............................. 1969
- **Support offered**........................... Supported

The Engadin Skimarathon is one of the most popular cross-country ski races in the world, held annually in the stunning Engadin Valley of Switzerland. Since 1969, the race has grown into one of the largest ski marathons globally, attracting skiers from all over the world, from elite athletes to recreational skiers. The Engadin Skimarathon takes place in one of Switzerland's most beautiful regions, with the race route running through picturesque villages and across frozen lakes. Over the years, the event has expanded to include shorter races and categories for skiers of all levels, making it accessible to a broad audience while maintaining its status as a key fixture in the international ski marathon circuit.

The race follows a relatively fast and scenic course through the Engadin Valley, starting in Maloja and finishing in S-chanf. The most notable feature of the course is the crossing of several frozen lakes, including Lake Sils and Lake St. Moritz, which offer wide, open sections where skiers can gain speed. The most challenging parts of the course are the narrow sections and the climb near the finish in S-chanf, which requires skiers to maintain their stamina after the long flat stretches. While the Engadin Skimarathon is not as technically demanding as some other ski marathons, its large number of participants can create crowded conditions, especially in the early stages of the race. Skiers must also adapt to the high altitude, as the race takes place at an elevation of around 1,800 meters (5,900 feet).

Entry is open to skiers of all levels, from elite athletes to recreational enthusiasts. There are no formal qualification requirements, making it an accessible event for anyone

You can find details about the Engadin Skimarathon on their official website:
https://www.engadin-skimarathon.ch/en/

DOG SLEDDING

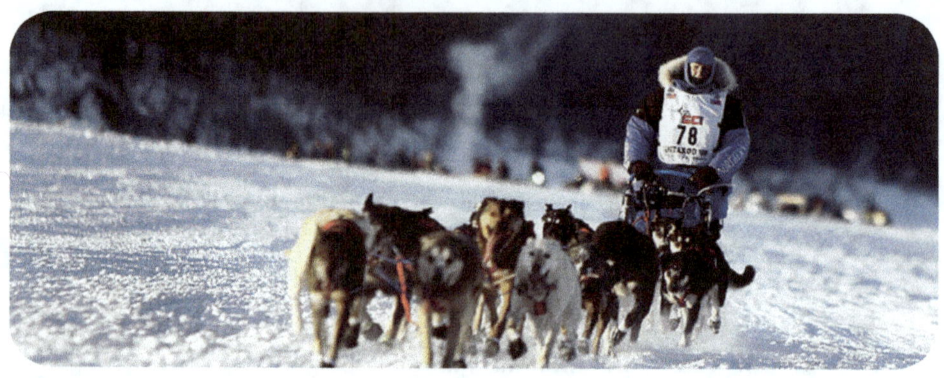

Dog sledding has a rich and storied history, deeply rooted in the survival strategies of indigenous peoples in the Arctic regions. For centuries, sled dogs were an essential mode of transportation in the harsh winter landscapes of Alaska, Canada, Siberia, and Greenland, where they played a crucial role in hunting, hauling supplies, and enabling communication between distant communities. The practice of dog sledding evolved from a necessity into a sport during the early 20th century, particularly after the famous 1925 serum run to Nome, Alaska, which showcased the incredible endurance and speed of sled dog teams. This historic event, in which dog teams relayed diphtheria antitoxin across 674 miles of treacherous terrain, inspired the creation of organized dog sledding races. Today, these races honor the legacy of those early sled teams, celebrating the unique bond between mushers and their dogs and the extraordinary endurance required to traverse some of the world's most challenging environments.

The first long-distance dog sledding race is widely recognized as the All-Alaska Sweepstakes, which began in 1908. This race, spanning 408 miles from Nome to Candle and back, set the stage for modern sled dog racing by establishing a competitive framework that challenged both mushers and their teams to cover vast distances under extreme conditions. The All-Alaska Sweepstakes ran annually until 1917 and was revived briefly in the 1980s, leaving a lasting legacy that influenced the development of other long-distance races. However, the most iconic of these is the Iditarod Trail Sled Dog Race, which first took place in 1973. The Iditarod was inspired by the 1925 serum run and sought to preserve the historic Iditarod Trail while promoting the sport of mushing. Spanning approximately 1,000 miles, the Iditarod quickly became the gold standard for endurance races, inspiring similar events across the globe.

As the sport of dog sledding has evolved, the races have become increasingly longer and more demanding, pushing the limits of both mushers and their dog teams. Initially, races were often short, designed to test speed over relatively brief distances.

However, as interest in the sport grew and the skills of mushers and their dogs improved, race organizers began to extend the courses, incorporating more challenging terrains and harsher environmental conditions. Today, races like the Yukon Quest and the Finnmarksløpet, both of which cover over 1,000 miles, represent the pinnacle of endurance racing, demanding not only speed but also extraordinary stamina and survival skills. The push to make races longer and tougher is driven by a combination of tradition, the desire to honor the historical routes of early mushers, and the competitive spirit of the sport, which continually seeks to test the boundaries of human and canine endurance.

The difficulty of dog sledding races is determined by a combination of factors, each of which tests the physical and mental limits of both mushers and their dogs. The sheer distance of these races, often stretching over 1,000 miles, requires incredible endurance, as teams must travel for days or even weeks through some of the most inhospitable environments on Earth. Harsh weather conditions, including extreme cold, blizzards, and gale-force winds, add to the challenge, making navigation difficult and increasing the risk of frostbite and hypothermia. The terrain itself can be unforgiving, with mushers navigating through dense forests, across frozen rivers, over mountain ranges, and along treacherous coastlines. Additionally, the isolation of the trail, with checkpoints often hundreds of miles apart, means that mushers must be self-reliant, capable of handling any emergencies that arise. These attributes—distance, weather, terrain, and isolation—combine to create races that are not only physically demanding but also mentally exhausting, requiring a deep bond of trust between mushers and their dogs and a relentless determination to reach the finish line.

IDITAROD TRAIL

- Location.................................... Alaska
- Time of year............................. March
- Approximate distance................. 1609km (1000 miles)
- Average time to finish................. 8 – 15 days
- Average number of entries.......... 50 – 60 teams
- Average cost to enter................... $4000 – $5000
- Year it started............................. 1973
- Support offered.......................... Semi-supported

The Iditarod Trail Sled Dog Race is one of the most iconic endurance events in the world, held annually in Alaska. Known as "The Last Great Race on Earth," the Iditarod was first run in 1973 as a way to preserve the historical Iditarod Trail and the tradition of sled dog mushing. The race commemorates the 1925 serum run to Nome, where dog sled teams delivered life-saving diphtheria serum during a deadly outbreak. Over the decades, the Iditarod has grown into a globally recognized event, attracting mushers from around the world who are drawn to the challenge of racing through Alaska's wilderness. The race begins in Anchorage and ends in Nome, covering approximately 1000 miles of some of the most remote terrain in North America.

The race alternates between the northern and southern routes, each presenting its own unique challenges. Mushers and their teams face extreme weather conditions, including blizzards, gale-force winds, and temperatures that can plummet to -50°F (-45°C). The race crosses the Alaska Range, including the treacherous Happy River Steps and the windy, barren expanses of the Yukon River. Mushers must also navigate the notorious "Farewell Burn," an area of charred forest, and the icy, unpredictable terrain of the Bering Sea coast.

To enter the Iditarod, mushers must meet strict qualification criteria, including completing a series of approved qualifying races that demonstrate their ability to handle long-distance sled dog racing in extreme conditions. The Iditarod places a strong emphasis on the welfare of the dogs, with mandatory veterinary checks before the race and at each checkpoint, ensuring that only the healthiest and fittest dogs participate.

You can find details about the Iditarod Trail race on their official website: https://iditarod.com/

FINNMARKSLØPET

- **Location**............................... Norway
- **Time of year**............................... March
- **Approximate distance**................. 1200km (745 miles)
- **Average time to finish**................. 5 – 7 days
- **Average number of entries**.......... 150 teams
- **Average cost to enter**................... $500 – $900
- **Year it started**............................. 1981
- **Support offered**........................... Semi-supported

Finnmarksløpet is the longest and northernmost sled dog race in Europe, and one of the premier events in the mushing world. Established in 1981, the race takes place in the Arctic wilderness of Finnmark, Norway, and has grown to become an iconic event for both mushers and dog teams. Originally conceived as a 500km race, Finnmarksløpet has expanded over the years to include a grueling 1200km category, making it a true test of endurance, strategy, and survival skills. The race attracts some of the best mushers from around the world, who come to compete in one of the most challenging environments on the planet. The race is deeply rooted in the culture of Northern Norway, celebrating the traditional way of life in the Arctic and the incredible bond between mushers and their dogs.

The course traverses the vast wilderness of Finnmark, Norway's largest and northernmost county. The race takes mushers through some of the most remote and inhospitable terrain in Europe, including frozen tundra, dense forests, and high mountain plateaus. The weather conditions can be extreme, with temperatures often dropping below -30°C (-22°F) and powerful Arctic winds creating whiteout conditions. The course is marked, but the isolation and vast distances between checkpoints add to the difficulty.

Entry is open to mushers who meet specific qualifications, particularly for the longer race categories. Mushers must demonstrate significant experience in long-distance sled dog racing, as well as the ability to care for and manage a team of sled dogs under extreme conditions. The race organizers require participants to complete a qualifying race and to provide evidence of their dogs' health and fitness.

You can find details about the Finnmarkslopet on their official website: https://www.finnmarkslopet.no/

KOBUK 440

- **Location**..................................... Alaska (United States)
- **Time of year**............................... April
- **Approximate distance**................ 708km (440 miles)
- **Average time to finish**................ 3 – 4 days
- **Average number of entries**.......... 15 – 20 teams
- **Average cost to enter**.................... $300 – $600
- **Year it started**............................. 1988
- **Support offered**........................... Semi-supported

The Kobuk 440 is one of Alaska's most challenging long-distance sled dog races, held annually in the Arctic region. Established in 1988, the race was designed to celebrate the mushing culture and the traditional skills of dog sledding in the Kobuk region. The Kobuk 440 has become a key event in the Alaskan mushing calendar, often serving as the final major race of the season. The race starts and finishes in the town of Kotzebue, making a loop through several remote villages, which are only accessible by dog sled or snowmobile during the winter months.

The Kobuk 440 course covers 440 miles of some of the most remote and challenging terrain in Alaska. The race begins in Kotzebue, a small town located above the Arctic Circle, and travels through a series of checkpoints, including Noorvik, Selawik, Ambler, and Shungnak, before looping back to Kotzebue. The Arctic weather conditions can be brutal, with temperatures frequently dropping below -30°F (-34°C) and strong winds creating whiteout conditions.

To participate in the Kobuk 440, mushers must have considerable experience in long-distance sled dog racing, particularly in extreme winter conditions. The race is open to seasoned mushers who can demonstrate their ability to manage a dog team over several days of racing through harsh and remote environments. Entrants are required to meet certain qualifications, including completing a qualifying race or providing proof of their experience in similar races.

You can find details about the Kobuk 440 on their official website:
http://www.kobuk440.com/

FEMUNDLØPET

- **Location**.. Norway
- **Time of year**.................................. February
- **Approximate distance**.................. 650km (404 miles)
- **Average time to finish**................. 4 – 6 days
- **Average number of entries**.......... 150 – 200 teams
- **Average cost to enter**.................... $250 – $700
- **Year it started**.............................. 1990
- **Support offered**........................... Semi-supported

Femundløpet is one of Europe's premier long-distance sled dog races, held annually in the snow-covered wilderness of Norway. Established in 1990, the race has become a major event in the mushing world, attracting top mushers from Norway and across the globe. The race is named after Femunden, the third-largest lake in Norway, around which much of the race is centered. Over the years, the event has grown to include multiple race distances, making it accessible to a range of competitors.

The course takes teams through some of the most beautiful yet challenging landscapes in Norway. The race begins and ends in the historic mining town of Røros, a UNESCO World Heritage site, and traverses the vast, snow-covered wilderness of the Femunden area. The longest race, F650, covers 650km of terrain through dense forests, frozen lakes, and high mountain plateaus. The weather in this region can be severe, with temperatures often dropping well below -20°C (-4°F), accompanied by strong winds and heavy snowfall. The race also involves navigating through long, isolated stretches where teams may not see another competitor for hours.

Entry is open to mushers who have sufficient experience in long-distance sled dog racing. For the F650 and F450 races, participants must have completed previous races of similar distances to ensure they are prepared for the course. The race organizers place a strong emphasis on the welfare of the dogs, requiring detailed health checks and ensuring that teams are properly equipped to handle the extreme conditions. Mushers must provide evidence of their dogs' fitness and training, and all teams are subject to rigorous veterinary inspections throughout the race.

You can find details about the Femundløpet on their official website:
https://www.femundlopet.no/v2/

CANADIAN CHALLENGE

- **Location**..................................... Canada
- **Time of year**............................... February
- **Approximate distance**................. 500km (311 miles)
- **Average time to finish**................. 3 – 5 days
- **Average number of entries**.......... 20 – 30 teams
- **Average cost to enter**................... $300 – $800
- **Year it started**............................. 1998
- **Support offered**........................... Semi-supported

The Canadian Challenge is one of Canada's premier long-distance sled dog races, taking place annually in the wilderness of Saskatchewan. Established in 1998, the race has grown in prominence and is now a key event on the mushing calendar, attracting teams from across Canada and beyond. The race offers multiple categories, with the longest being a 500km trek that challenges mushers and their teams to navigate the remote and often harsh winter conditions of northern Canada.

The course covering 500km, starts in Prince Albert and follows a route that includes remote checkpoints such as La Ronge and Missinipe before returning to the starting point. The terrain is varied, with long stretches through dense forests, over frozen lakes, and across open plains. The weather can be extremely cold, with temperatures often dropping below -30°C (-22°F), and conditions can change rapidly, with blizzards and high winds making navigation and progress difficult.

Participation in the Canadian Challenge is open to experienced mushers who have the necessary skills and preparation to complete a long-distance race in extreme winter conditions. For the 500km race, mushers must have prior experience in similar long-distance events or provide evidence of their capability to handle the challenges of the race.

You can find details about Canadian Challenge on their official website:
https://canadianchallenge.com/

LA GRANDE ODYSSÉE

- **Location**................................... France & Switzerland
- **Time of year**.............................. January
- **Approximate distance**................. 400km (250 miles)
- **Average time to finish**............... 10 – 12 days
- **Average number of entries**.......... 20 – 25 teams
- **Average cost to enter**................... 2005
- **Year it started**............................. $1000 – $2000
- **Support offered**........................... Semi-supported

La Grande Odyssée is one of the most prestigious and challenging sled dog races in the world, held annually in the French and Swiss Alps. Since its inception in 2005, the race has become a highlight of the winter sports calendar, attracting some of the best mushers from around the globe. Designed to showcase the beauty of the Alpine regions while testing the endurance and skills of both mushers and their dog teams, La Grande Odyssée is renowned for its demanding course, which traverses high-altitude landscapes with steep climbs and descents. The race has grown in stature over the years, now serving as a key event for the mushing community in Europe, combining the sport's traditions with the unique challenges posed by the Alps.

The race route includes some of the most challenging terrains in Europe, with high-altitude passes, deep snow, and steep mountain trails. The altitude, which can reach over 2,000 meters (6,560 feet), adds to the physical demands on both the dogs and the mushers. Each stage of the race is meticulously planned to challenge the teams' endurance, navigation skills, and ability to maintain the health and performance of their dogs under extreme conditions.

Participation in La Grande Odyssée is limited to experienced mushers who have demonstrated their ability to handle long-distance sled dog races. The entry criteria include a selection process where mushers must provide evidence of their experience, particularly in high-altitude and mountainous environments. The race organizers also require detailed information about the health and conditioning of the dog teams. Mushers must also adhere to strict rules regarding the welfare of their dogs, with regular veterinary checks and mandatory rest periods to ensure the safety and well-being of the teams.

You can find details about the La Grande Odyssée on their official website:
https://www.grandeodyssee.com/en/

SKI MOUNTAINEERING

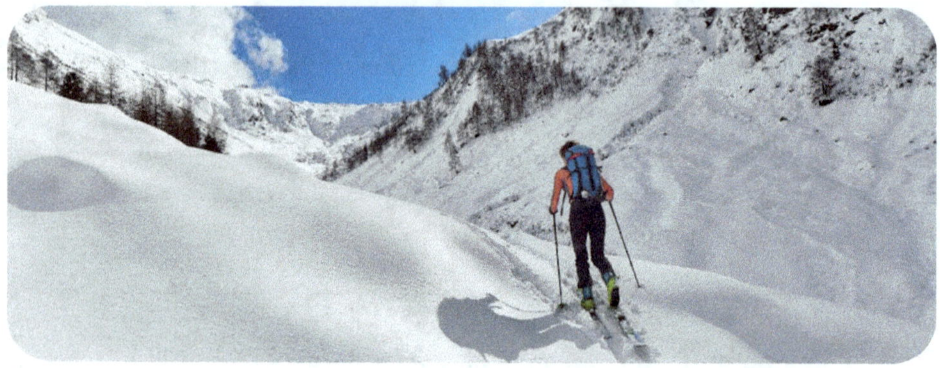

Ski mountaineering racing, also known as skimo, is a demanding sport that combines alpine skiing with mountaineering. In racing, competitors ascend and descend mountainous terrain using a combination of specialized equipment, including climbing skins for the ascents and ski bindings that can switch between ski and walk modes. Races are designed to test both endurance and technical prowess, often including sections of steep climbing, challenging descents, and navigation through variable snow conditions. The courses are typically set in mountainous environments and can range from short sprints to multi-hour events covering significant vertical gain and distance. Ski mountaineering racing requires athletes to efficiently manage their energy, skills, and equipment to complete the course in the shortest time while overcoming the physical and environmental challenges of the terrain.

Ski mountaineering has its roots in traditional alpine skiing and mountaineering practices. The sport's origins can be traced back to the late 19th and early 20th centuries, as alpine enthusiasts began combining skiing with mountain ascents. The formalization of ski mountaineering racing began in the 1980s in Europe, particularly in the French Alps, where enthusiasts sought to combine the thrill of skiing with the challenge of mountain climbing. The International Ski Mountaineering Federation (ISMF), founded in 1988, played a crucial role in organizing and standardizing the sport at an international level. Since then, ski mountaineering has gained popularity globally, with organised races becoming a central feature of the sport, leading to the inclusion of ski mountaineering as a demonstration sport in the Winter Olympics in 2026.

The evolution of long endurance races in ski mountaineering began with events designed to push the limits of physical and technical endurance. One of the earliest notable long-distance races is the Patrouille des Glaciers, first held in 1943 in Switzerland. Initially a military training event, it evolved into a major competitive race, covering a challenging course from Zermatt to Verbier.

The race has since become a prestigious event in the ski mountaineering calendar, featuring a demanding course that tests participants' endurance, navigation, and ability to handle extreme mountain conditions. These early long-distance races set a precedent for the development of endurance events in the sport, establishing benchmarks for distance and difficulty.

Ski mountaineering races have become increasingly challenging due to advances in technology, evolving race formats, and growing competitive standards. Modern races often feature longer distances, greater vertical ascents, and more technical terrain than their predecessors. The advent of advanced equipment, such as lighter and more efficient skis, bindings, and climbing skins, has enabled athletes to tackle more demanding courses at higher speeds. Additionally, race organizers are incorporating new formats, such as multi-day stage races and complex navigation challenges, to further test competitors' endurance and skills. The increasing level of competition, with more elite athletes and sophisticated training techniques, has also contributed to the rising difficulty of races, making them more physically demanding.

The difficulty of ski mountaineering races is driven by a combination of physical, environmental, and technical challenges. Physically, athletes must endure prolonged periods of exertion, managing the demands of both climbing and descending mountainous terrain. The environmental factors, including unpredictable weather, variable snow conditions, and high altitudes require competitors to adapt their strategies and techniques in real-time.

PIERRA MENTA

- **Location**.................................... France
- **Time of year**............................. March
- **Approximate distance**................. 100km (62 miles)
- **Average time to finish**................. 4 days (4 – 6 hours per day)
- **Average number of entries**.......... 400 participants
- **Average cost to enter**................... $300 – $500
- **Year it started**............................. 1986
- **Support offered**........................... Supported

The Pierra Menta is one of the most challenging ski mountaineering races in the world. Held annually in the French Alps in the Beaufortain Massif, the race has been a key event in the international ski mountaineering calendar since it was first organized in 1986. The Pierra Menta is part of the "La Grande Course" circuit, which includes the most iconic ski mountaineering races across Europe. The event is unique in that it is a team race, with two-person teams required to stay together throughout the entire race, adding an extra layer of strategy and cooperation to the competition.

The Pierra Menta course is spread over four days, covering approximately 100km with a staggering 10,000 meters of vertical gain. Each day, teams face a series of steep ascents and technical descents, navigating exposed ridges, narrow couloirs, and vast snowfields. The race requires a high level of technical skill in ski mountaineering, including the ability to climb efficiently with skins, transition quickly between climbing and descending, and handle challenging downhill sections in often variable snow conditions. The course is known for its spectacular yet demanding terrain, with some stages including knife-edge ridges where competitors must use crampons and ropes. The weather in the high Alps can be unpredictable, adding another layer of difficulty to the race. The combination of long distances, massive elevation changes, and technical challenges makes the Pierra Menta one of the toughest races in the sport, attracting only the most experienced and fit ski mountaineers.

Entry into the Pierra Menta is highly competitive, and the race typically attracts the best ski mountaineers from around the world. Only those with significant experience in ski mountaineering races are encouraged to enter.

You can find details about Pierra Menta on their official website: https://pierramenta.com/

TOUR DU RUTOR

- **Location**.. Italy
- **Time of year**................................... March
- **Approximate distance**................. 75km (46.6 miles)
- **Average time to finish**................ 3 days (4 – 6 hours per day)
- **Average number of entries**.......... 700 participants
- **Average cost to enter**.................... $300 – $500
- **Year it started**.............................. 1933
- **Support offered**........................... Supported

The Tour du Rutor is one of the most prestigious ski mountaineering races in the world, held biennially in the Aosta Valley of Italy. Originally started in 1933, the race was revived in 1995 as part of the modern ski mountaineering competition circuit. It is now part of the "La Grande Course" series, which includes the most iconic ski mountaineering races in Europe. The race is known for its breathtaking alpine scenery, technical difficulty, and the intense competition it attracts. Teams of two compete over three days, tackling steep climbs, technical descents, and exposed ridges.

The Tour du Rutor course spans approximately 75km over three days, with a total vertical gain of around 7,000 meters. Each stage of the race features a mix of steep ascents, technical descents, and long traverses across glaciers and exposed ridges. The course requires a high level of technical skill, including proficiency in using crampons, ropes, and other mountaineering equipment. The altitude, which often exceeds 3,000 meters, adds to the physical demands, as participants must cope with the effects of reduced oxygen levels. The weather in the high Alps can be unpredictable, with potential for strong winds, low temperatures, and snowstorms.

Entry into the Tour du Rutor is highly competitive, with spots typically filled by teams with significant experience in ski mountaineering. Each team consists of two members who must stay together throughout the race.

You can find details about the Tour du Rutor on their official website:
https://tourdurutor.com/en

ANDORRA SKIMO 10

- **Location**...................................... Andorra
- **Time of year**............................... February
- **Approximate distance**................. 70km (43.5 miles)
- **Average time to finish**................. 2 days (8 – 10 hours per day)
- **Average number of entries**.......... 450 participants
- **Average cost to enter**................... $100
- **Year it started**............................. 2016
- **Support offered**........................... Semi-supported

The Andorra Skimo race series started in 2016 as part of a vision to establish a comprehensive ski mountaineering challenge that spans Andorra's winter terrain. Originally beginning with the Skimo 6, which covered six high-altitude mountain refuges, the race was expanded to include the Skimo 10 in 2018. This extension brought the total distance to approximately 70 km, offering participants a more challenging, multi-stage course. It has quickly grown in popularity, attracting both professional and amateur skiers who want to race in the Pyrenees.

The Skimo 10 takes participants through some of Andorra's most iconic high-altitude locations. The race starts at Naturlandia in Sant Julià de Lòria and covers two stages. The first stage takes racers to Grau Roig, navigating through six mountain refuges and scenic areas such as the Estany de la Nou, the Illa, and the Vall del Madriu-Perafita-Claror (a UNESCO World Heritage site). The second stage continues from Grau Roig to Ordino-Arcalís, making the course both physically demanding and visually stunning. The race is known for its challenging climbs, steep descents, and views of the Pyrenean landscape.

To participate, racers must compete in teams of two or three. There are no specific pre-qualification requirements, but entrants should be well-versed in ski mountaineering and prepared for the physical and technical demands of the race. Participants are required to have the necessary equipment for safe travel in the mountains, including avalanche safety gear, appropriate skis, skins, and other essential mountaineering gear. The race also contributes points towards the Andorra Mountain Skiing Cup, making it valuable for competitive skiers.

You can find details about Andorra Skimo 10 on their official website: https://www.andorraskimo.com/en/skimo10

THE GRAND TRAVERSE

- **Location**..................................... Colorado (United States)
- **Time of year**.............................. March
- **Approximate distance**................. 64km (40 miles)
- **Average time to finish**................ 8 – 16 hours
- **Average number of entries**.......... 400 participants
- **Average cost to enter**.................. $400 – $500 per team
- **Year it started**............................ 1998
- **Support offered**.......................... Supported

The Grand Traverse is a legendary backcountry ski race that spans the Elk Mountains of Colorado, from Crested Butte to Aspen. Established in 1998, this race was inspired by the traditional European ski mountaineering races and is designed to test the endurance, navigation skills, and teamwork of participants as they traverse some of Colorado's most challenging and remote terrain. The race begins at midnight, adding an extra layer of difficulty as competitors must navigate through the night, often in harsh winter conditions. The Grand Traverse is unique in its combination of ski mountaineering, endurance racing, and backcountry survival, making it one of the most challenging and respected races in North America.

The race requires participants to climb over 6,800 feet of vertical gain, including a crossing of the 12,303-foot Star Pass. Because the race begins at midnight, participants must navigate much of the course in the dark, relying on headlamps, maps, and GPS devices. The high altitude and unpredictable mountain weather, which can range from snowstorms to freezing temperatures, add to the challenge. Teams must also carry mandatory survival gear, including a bivy sack, stove, and extra clothing, in case of emergency.

Entry into The Grand Traverse is open to teams of two, and participants must have significant experience in backcountry skiing and be in excellent physical condition. The race is demanding, and while there are no formal qualification requirements, it is recommended that participants have experience in similar long-distance ski mountaineering races or extensive backcountry travel.

You can find details about The Grand Traverse on their official website: https://thegrandtraverse.org/ski/

PATROUILLE DES GLACIERS

- **Location**.. Switzerland
- **Time of year**................................. April
- **Approximate distance**.................. 57.5km (35.7 miles)
- **Average time to finish**................. 10 – 16 hours
- **Average number of entries**.......... 4000 participants
- **Average cost to enter**................... $150 – $300
- **Year it started**............................. 1943
- **Support offered**........................... Supported

The Patrouille des Glaciers (PDG) is one of the most iconic ski mountaineering races in the world, held biennially in the Swiss Alps. The race was originally conceived in 1943 by the Swiss Army as a way to test the endurance and skills of its soldiers during World War II. Today, it has evolved into a major international event that attracts elite athletes and mountaineers from around the world. The PDG is a team event, with each team consisting of three members who must stay together throughout the race.

The Patrouille des Glaciers offers two routes: the longer Zermatt-Verbier route (57.5km) and the shorter Arolla-Verbier route (29.6km). Both routes take participants through the heart of the Swiss Alps, traversing glaciers, high mountain passes, and steep climbs, often at altitudes exceeding 3,000 meters (9,800 feet). The course is renowned for its technical difficulty, with teams navigating crevassed glaciers, exposed ridges, and long, grueling ascents. The weather in the high Alps can be unpredictable, with conditions ranging from clear skies to blizzards and sub-zero temperatures. The race requires not only excellent physical conditioning but also strong mountaineering skills, as participants must be capable of using crampons, ropes, and other technical equipment.

Entry into the Patrouille des Glaciers is highly competitive, with spots typically allocated through a lottery system due to the high demand. Each team must consist of three members who have demonstrated their ability to handle the rigors of ski mountaineering. Teams are required to undergo a strict qualification process, including proving their experience in high-altitude, long-distance ski mountaineering races.

You can find details about the Patrouille des Glaciers on their official website: https://www.pdg.ch/en/

- **Location**.............................. Italy
- **Time of year**........................... April
- **Approximate distance**.............. 45km (28 miles)
- **Average time to finish**.............. 5 – 6 hours
- **Average number of entries**.......... 900 participants
- **Average cost to enter**.................. $600 – $700 per team
- **Year it started**........................... 1933
- **Support offered**.......................... Supported

The Trofeo Mezzalama is one of the most prestigious ski mountaineering races in the world. It is part of the "La Grande Course" series, which includes the most iconic ski mountaineering races in Europe. The Trofeo Mezzalama is named after Ottorino Mezzalama, an early pioneer of alpine skiing, and was first held in 1933. The race is held biennially in the Monte Rosa massif, the second-highest mountain range in the Alps. It is a true test of endurance, skill, and teamwork, taking place at high altitudes in some of the most rugged and beautiful terrain in the Alps. The race covers a distance of approximately 45km and includes challenging ascents, technical descents, and sections where participants must use ropes and crampons. The race is unique in that it takes place entirely at high altitude, with much of the course above 3,000 meters, making it a demanding challenge for even the most experienced mountaineers.

The Trofeo Mezzalama course is known for its extreme difficulty due to its high altitude, technical terrain, and challenging weather conditions. The race starts in Cervinia and finishes in Gressoney-La-Trinité, crossing the Monte Rosa massif. The route includes climbs to the summits of Castor (4,228 meters) and Naso del Lyskamm (4,272 meters), requiring participants to traverse glaciers, steep ridges, and exposed sections. The high altitude makes the race particularly demanding, as the thin air reduces oxygen levels and increases the risk of altitude sickness. The technical nature of the course requires participants to be proficient in using crampons, ice axes and ropes.

Entry into the Trofeo Mezzalama is highly competitive, and teams are selected based on their experience and past performances in similar events. Each team consists of three members who must stay together throughout the race.

You can find details about the Trofeo Mezzalama on their official website: https://www.trofeomezzalama.it/

ADAMELLO SKI RAID

- **Location**..................................... Italy
- **Time of year**............................... April
- **Approximate distance**................. 43km (27 miles)
- **Average time to finish**................ 5 – 8 hours
- **Average number of entries**.......... 600 participants
- **Average cost to enter**................... $250 – $400
- **Year it started**............................. 2006
- **Support offered**........................... Supported

The Adamello Ski Raid is a prestigious and challenging ski mountaineering race held in the Adamello-Presanella Alps in northern Italy. Established in 2006, the race has quickly gained a reputation as one of the most demanding and scenic events in the ski mountaineering world. It is part of the "La Grande Course" series, which includes some of the most iconic and difficult races in Europe. The Adamello Ski Raid is known for its breathtaking course through the rugged and snowy terrain of the Adamello Massif, an area steeped in history, particularly from World War I, when the region was the site of intense mountain warfare. The race attracts top athletes from around the world who come to test their endurance, skill, and teamwork in this challenging alpine environment.

The Adamello Ski Raid course covers approximately 43km with a staggering vertical gain of around 4,000 meters. The race starts in the town of Ponte di Legno and takes participants through the heart of the Adamello Massif, crossing glaciers, steep ridges, and high-altitude passes. The course includes several challenging ascents, with some climbs reaching over 3,000 meters above sea level. The terrain is highly technical, requiring participants to use crampons, ropes, and other mountaineering equipment, particularly when crossing exposed ridges and steep couloirs. The high altitude, combined with the physical demands of the course and the potential for severe weather, makes the Adamello Ski Raid one of the toughest races in the sport

Entry into the Adamello Ski Raid is highly competitive, with teams selected based on their experience and past performances in similar events. Each team consists of two members who must stay together throughout the race.

You can find details about Adamello Ski Raid on their official website: https://www.adamelloskiraid.com/

SELLARONDA SKI MARATHON

- **Location**... Italy
- **Time of year**................................. March
- **Approximate distance**................. 42km (26 miles)
- **Average time to finish**................ 3 – 5 hours
- **Average number of entries**.......... 1300 participants
- **Average cost to enter**................... $150 – $200
- **Year it started**............................. 1995
- **Support offered**........................... Supported

The Sellaronda Ski Marathon is one of the most prestigious and exciting ski mountaineering races in the world, held annually in the breathtaking Dolomites of Italy. Established in 1995, the race has quickly become a key event in the ski mountaineering calendar, attracting top athletes and enthusiastic amateurs alike. The Sellaronda is a night race, adding an extra layer of challenge and excitement as participants navigate the course by headlamp. The race follows a circular route around the Sella massif, passing through four famous Dolomite passes—Passo Pordoi, Passo Sella, Passo Gardena, and Passo Campolongo—and crossing through four picturesque villages: Canazei, Corvara, Arabba, and Selva di Val Gardena. The combination of stunning scenery, technical challenges, and the unique atmosphere of a night race makes the Sellaronda Ski Marathon a must-do for any serious ski mountaineer.

The race has a total vertical gain of around 2,700 meters. It starts and finishes in one of the four main villages (the starting point rotates each year), and participants must complete the loop around the Sella massif. The course includes a mix of steep climbs, technical descents, and long traverses across the Dolomite passes, requiring a high level of fitness, technical skill, and strategic pacing. The fact that the race takes place at night adds a significant challenge, as participants must navigate the course with limited visibility, relying on their headlamps and knowledge of the terrain.

Entry into the Sellaronda Ski Marathon is open to teams of two, and the race is highly popular, often filling up quickly after registration opens. There are no formal qualification requirements, but participants should have significant experience in ski mountaineering and be in excellent physical condition.

You can find details about the Sellaronda Ski Marathon on their official website: https://www.sellaronda.it/en/

ALTITOY-TERNUA

- **Location**... France & Spain
- **Time of year**................................. February
- **Approximate distance**.................. 45km (28 miles)
- **Average time to finish**................. 6 – 10 hours (2 days)
- **Average number of entries**.......... 500 participants
- **Average cost to enter**................... $100 – $150
- **Year it started**.............................. 2008
- **Support offered**........................... Supported

The Altitoy-Ternua is one of the most challenging skimo races in the Pyrenees. It has been held annually since 2008, and is part of the prestigious "La Grande Course" series, which includes some of the most iconic ski mountaineering races in Europe. The Altitoy-Ternua is known for its scenery and tough course, which spans the Pyrenees mountain range between France and Spain, near the La Mongie and Barèges ski areas. The race typically takes place over two days, with competitors forming teams of two.

The Altitoy-Ternua course covers roughly 45km over two days, with significant vertical gains of around 4,000-5,000 meters in total. The race route winds through the terrain of the Pyrenees, offering a combination of steep ascents, technical descents, and long traverses across snowy ridges and glaciers. The course often includes challenging passages, such as narrow couloirs and exposed ridgelines, where competitors must use crampons, ropes, and other mountaineering equipment. Additionally, the weather in the Pyrenees can be highly variable, with the possibility of snowstorms, high winds, and poor visibility, further increasing the difficulty. The combination of technical skiing, long ascents, and unpredictable weather makes the Altitoy-Ternua one of the most difficult and rewarding ski mountaineering races in the Pyrenees.

Entry into the Altitoy-Ternua is open to teams of two who're required to compete together throughout the race. While there are no formal qualification requirements, participants should have significant experience in high-altitude ski mountaineering and be comfortable with technical terrain.

You can find details about the Altitoy-Ternua on their official website:
https://www.altitoy-skialpinisme.com/en

CHAPTER 4 - WATER SPORTS

In Chapter 4, we delve into some of the toughest endurance sports in the world that take place on or in the water. These sports encompass a wide variety of challenges, each presenting its own unique demands and requiring an extraordinary level of physical and mental endurance. We start with swimming, a sport that truly pits the athlete against the elements. In open water swimming, competitors must battle through potentially hazardous conditions such as cold temperatures, strong currents, and unpredictable weather. The endurance required to maintain a steady pace over long distances is immense, as swimmers push their bodies to the limits in an environment where the only resistance comes from nature itself. Moving on to sports like kayaking and paddleboarding, we see how athletes rely on their own strength and stamina to propel themselves across stretches of water. These sports demand not only physical power but also a great deal of technical skill. Every stroke counts and the ability to remain focused and efficient in movement is crucial. Finally, we will explore sailing, where athletes must use their knowledge and understanding of the elements to their advantage. Unlike swimming or paddling, where physical exertion is the primary focus, sailing requires the wind to propel their boats forward and the endurance required in sailing comes not only from the physical demands of managing the boat but also from the mental stamina needed to make quick, calculated decisions over long periods, often with little rest.

All these water-based sports hold a significant place among the list of the world's toughest endurance races. Whether you're drawn to the primal challenge of swimming against the current, the isolation of paddling across open waters, or the strategic mastery of sailing, these endurance sports offer a glimpse into the extreme lengths humans will go to test their limits. As we explore these incredible feats, we gain a deeper appreciation for the athletes who brave the elements and push themselves beyond what most would consider possible.

SWIMMING

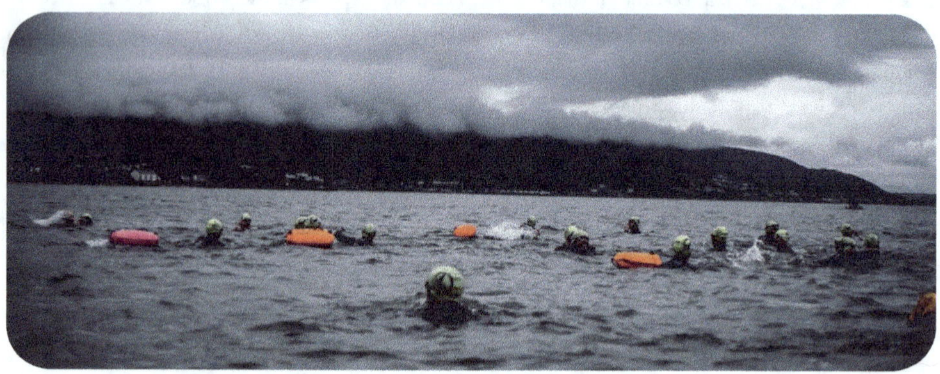

Open water swimming involves racing in natural bodies of water such as lakes, rivers, and oceans, rather than in a controlled pool environment. This discipline requires athletes to navigate varying conditions including waves, currents, and temperature fluctuations. Unlike pool races, which are often confined to standard distances and well-defined lanes, open water races are more dynamic and can vary greatly in course layout and length. Participants must contend with the challenges of sighting along with managing their energy and technique amidst unpredictable water conditions.

The history of open water swimming is varied, with roots extending back to ancient times. Historical accounts and mythology from cultures around the world, including the Greeks, Romans, and Egyptians, highlight the significance of swimming in natural waters. One of the earliest recorded open water swims was the legendary swim of Leander, who is said to have swum across the Hellespont (modern-day Dardanelles) to be with his lover, Hero. However, organised open water swimming as a sport began to take shape in the 19th century. The English Channel swim, first completed by Captain Matthew Webb in 1875, marked a pivotal moment in the sport's history, establishing the benchmark for endurance swimming across challenging distances. The early 20th century saw the introduction of formal marathon swims, and by the mid-century, open water events began to gain prominence with the establishment of competitive open water races and the inclusion of marathon swimming in the Olympic Games.

Following the English channel swim by Captain Matthew Webb in 1875, the early 20th century saw the rise of other significant long-distance swims, including notable marathon swims in locations such as the Strait of Gibraltar and across various lakes and rivers. The evolution of open water swimming has led to increasingly challenging races, driven by advancements in both technology and training. Advances in wetsuit technology and other equipment have enabled swimmers to compete in colder waters and handle more extreme environments, though they also add their own set of challenges.

Training methodologies have become more sophisticated, incorporating sports science and data analytics to enhance performance and adapt to the varied conditions of open water. The introduction of ultra-endurance events, such as 25 km or even 48-hour swims, demonstrates the sport's shift towards ever more demanding challenges.

Several factors contribute to the difficulty of open water swimming races, each adding unique challenges compared to pool swimming. The most prominent factor is the variable nature of the environment. Swimmers must contend with unpredictable water conditions such as waves, currents, and varying temperatures, which can significantly impact their performance and safety. Navigational challenges also play a crucial role; swimmers need to use landmarks or floating buoys to stay on course, which can be particularly demanding in open water with no clear boundaries.

20 BRIDGES SWIM

- **Location**.. New York City (United States)
- **Time of year**................................ July
- **Approximate distance**.................. 45.9km (28.5miles)
- **Average time to finish**................. 6 – 9 hours
- **Average number of entries**.......... 20 – 30 participants
- **Average cost to enter**................... $2500 – $3500
- **Year it started**............................. 1982
- **Support offered**........................... Supported

The 20 Bridges Swim, formerly known as the Manhattan Island Marathon Swim, is a prestigious open-water swimming event that involves circumnavigating Manhattan Island. The event, renamed to highlight the 20 bridges it passes under, was officially organized under this name in 2016 by New York Open Water. It attracts experienced marathon swimmers from around the world and is part of the Triple Crown of Open Water Swimming, which also includes the English Channel and the Catalina Channel swims.

Circumnavigating Manhattan Island presents swimmers with a challenging 28.5 mile course through varied water conditions. The swim starts and ends at Battery Park, with swimmers navigating the strong and unpredictable currents of the East River, Harlem River, and Hudson River. The difficulty of the race is compounded by factors such as changing tides, boat traffic, and potential debris in the water. Furthermore, water quality and weather conditions can vary, adding to the challenge of this marathon swim.

Entry into the 20 Bridges Swim is highly selective, designed for seasoned marathon swimmers with proven experience in long-distance open water events. Applicants are required to submit a detailed swimming resume that includes past marathon swims and times, demonstrating their capability to complete the swim within the stipulated time frame. Health certifications and a qualifying swim are also typically required to ensure that participants can safely handle the demanding conditions of the course. Due to the limited number of slots available, the selection process is competitive, prioritising swimmers with strong credentials and experience in similar conditions.

You can find details about the 20 Bridges Swim on their official website:
https://www.nyopenwater.org/20-bridges-swim/

CAPRI-NAPOLI

- **Location**...................................... Italy
- **Time of year**.............................. September
- **Approximate distance**................. 36km (22.4 miles)
- **Average time to finish**................ 6 – 9 hours
- **Average number of entries**.......... 50 participants
- **Average cost to enter**.................. $500 – $1000
- **Year it started**............................ 1954
- **Support offered**.......................... Supported

The Capri-Napoli marathon swim is one of the most renowned long-distance open water swimming competitions in the world. Originally part of the global professional marathon swimming circuit until 1992, it was reintroduced in 1999 as an annual event attracting elite open water swimmers. The race covers the scenic stretch of water between the picturesque island of Capri and the coastal city of Naples, a stretch of the sea famous for marathon swimming.

During the 36km swimmers face multiple challenges, including navigating through potentially choppy waters, dealing with changing currents, and maintaining a high level of physical performance in a saltwater environment. The mental stamina required to sustain focus and energy across many hours in the open sea makes this race particularly tough, even for the most experienced swimmers.

Entry to the Capri-Napoli swim is highly competitive, typically reserved for experienced and elite open-water swimmers. Potential participants must submit an application including their swimming resume, which should demonstrate considerable experience in long-distance open water events and a history of competitive performance. Proof of recent completion of similarly demanding swims is often required to assess the swimmer's capability and endurance. Safety is a priority, so each swimmer must organise their own support boat and crew, which is essential for navigation, feeding, and emergency situations.

You can find details about Capri-Napoli swim on their official website:
https://web.caprinapoli.com/

LAKE ZURICH SWIM

- **Location**.. Switzerland
- **Time of year**.................................. August
- **Approximate distance**.................. 26.4km (16.4 miles)
- **Average time to finish**................. 6 – 12 hours
- **Average number of entries**.......... 25 – 30 participants
- **Average cost to enter**................... $450 – $650
- **Year it started**............................. 1987
- **Support offered**........................... Supported

The Sri Chinmoy Marathon Lake Zurich Swim is one of the most prestigious open-water swimming events in Europe. First held in 1987, the race was established by the Sri Chinmoy Marathon Team, known for organizing endurance events worldwide. The Lake Zurich Swim is a point-to-point race covering the entire length of Lake Zurich, from the town of Rapperswil at the southern end to Zurich at the northern end. Over the years, the event has grown in popularity and now attracts elite open-water swimmers from around the globe who are eager to test their endurance in one of Switzerland's most beautiful and serene settings.

The course begins in Rapperswil and finishes in Zurich, taking swimmers through some of the most picturesque landscapes in Switzerland. Swimmers must contend with fluctuating water temperatures, which can range from 18°C to 24°C (64°F to 75°F), and unpredictable weather, which can bring wind, rain, and choppy waters.

Entry into the swim is selective, with a rigorous application process designed to ensure that only experienced marathon swimmers participate. Prospective participants must submit a detailed swimming resume, highlighting previous marathon swims, preferably of distances 20km (12.4 miles) or more. Applicants may also be required to provide references from recognised swim officials or coaches who can attest to their ability. All swimmers must provide their own support crew, typically consisting of a kayaker or small boat team, to assist with navigation and feeding.

You can find details about Lake Zurich swim on their official website:
https://ch.srichinmoyraces.org/

PORT TO PUB

- **Location**.. Australia
- **Time of year**................................. March
- **Approximate distance**................. 25km (15.5miles)
- **Average time to finish**................ 6 – 10 hours
- **Average number of entries**.......... 100 participants
- **Average cost to enter**................... $400
- **Year it started**............................. 2016
- **Support offered**........................... Supported

The Port to Pub Ultra Distance swim was introduced to offer a more challenging version of the standard Port to Pub swim, which was established in 2016. The ultra distance attracts both local and international swimmers who are looking to push their limits beyond the traditional marathon swimming distance, making it a prestigious and competitive event in the global open-water community.

The 25km ultra distance course of the Port to Pub swim is designed to be a significant challenge, extending the standard route by over 5km into deeper and more open waters where swimmers often face stronger currents and potentially rougher sea conditions. The course's added length increases the demand on swimmers' endurance and exposes them to fluctuating conditions for a longer period, which can affect their speed and energy levels drastically.

To participate in the Port to Pub Ultra Distance event, swimmers must meet entry requirements to ensure they are capable of handling the extreme demands of the swim. This includes providing proof of completing a qualifying swim, which would typically be a 10km open water swim within a specific timeframe prior to the race day. Additionally, entrants must be aged 18 years or older and are expected to have a history of competing in similar long-distance open water events. Safety is paramount, so each swimmer is required to be accompanied by a support paddler and a support boat equipped with essential safety and communication gear, ensuring immediate assistance is available if needed.

You can find details about the Port to Pub swim on their official website:
https://porttopub.com.au/

VIDÖSTERNSIMMET

- **Location**..................................... Sweden
- **Time of year**................................ August
- **Approximate distance**.................. 21km (13 miles)
- **Average time to finish**................. 6 – 8 hours
- **Average number of entries**.......... 100 – 150 participants
- **Average cost to enter**.................. $100
- **Year it started**............................ 2011
- **Support offered**........................... Supported

Vidösternsimmet is Sweden's longest open-water swimming competition and has been challenging swimmers since 2011. It takes place in Lake Vidöstern, near Värnamo, and was started to provide a rigorous test of endurance for open water swimmers. The race has grown in popularity, drawing participants from across Scandinavia and beyond, attracted by the challenge of conquering one of the most demanding swims in northern Europe. The event not only tests physical endurance but also celebrates the beauty of the Swedish landscape.

The course of Vidösternsimmet spans 21.5km through Lake Vidöstern, known for its cold and often choppy waters. The length of the course is a significant challenge in itself, compounded by the variable weather conditions which can include wind and rain, which affect water surface conditions and visibility.

Entry to Vidösternsimmet is open to experienced open-water swimmers who can demonstrate their ability to handle long distances in potentially cold and challenging conditions. Applicants may be required to provide evidence of having completed similar distances in open water, ensuring that all participants are adequately prepared for the demands of the swim. Safety is paramount, so each swimmer must follow strict guidelines regarding support craft, either accompanying themselves with a kayak or a support boat. All participants must adhere to the event's safety protocols, including wearing a wetsuit unless they have special authorization to swim without one based on their experience and past performance in similar conditions.

You can find details about the Vidösternsimmet on their official website:
https://vidosternsimmet.com/

THE ROTTNEST CHANNEL SWIM

- **Location**.................................... Australia
- **Time of year**.............................. February
- **Approximate distance**................. 19.7km (12.3 miles)
- **Average time to finish**................ 4 – 8 hours
- **Average number of entries**.......... 2500 participants
- **Average cost to enter**.................. $250
- **Year it started**............................. 1991
- **Support offered**.......................... Supported

The Rottnest Channel Swim is one of Australia's most iconic open water swimming events, annually attracting thousands of swimmers from across the globe. The event began in 1991, inspired by earlier unofficial crossings, and has grown significantly in popularity since. It is now one of the largest open water swimming events in the world. The race showcases the beautiful coastline of Western Australia, which makes it a beloved fixture in the local sporting calendar.

The course of the Rottnest Channel Swim is a straight line from Cottesloe Beach to Rottnest Island, but don't let its straightforward path fool you, the swim is challenging due to a variety of factors. The distance itself is the initial obstacle, combined with potential strong currents, wind conditions, and water temperatures that can make the swim particularly harsh. Swimmers may also encounter marine life, such as jellyfish and seaweed, adding to the physical and mental challenge.

Entry into the Rottnest Channel Swim is open to solo swimmers and teams, with different categories based on age and team size. Solo swimmers must qualify by completing a qualifying swim of 10km in a specific time based on age and gender, conducted within a year of the event. This qualification ensures that all participants have demonstrated the ability to complete long-distance open water swims safely. Team members are not required to qualify but must demonstrate proficiency in swimming. All participants must have a support boat and a skipper, and solo swimmers are also required to have a support paddler to accompany them, ensuring safety and compliance with event regulations.

You can find details about Rottnest Channel Swim on their official website:
https://rottnestchannelswim.com.au/

KAYAKING

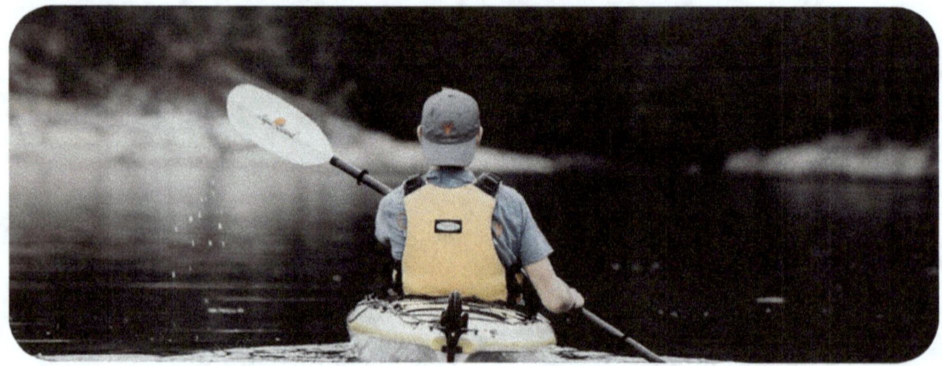

Kayaking is a sport that involves athletes propelling a kayak or canoe through water using a double-bladed paddle. Marathon or long-distance kayaking races can span long distances and often take place on rivers, lakes, or coastal waters, requiring a combination of endurance, technique, and strategic planning. In all these formats, the primary goal is to achieve the fastest time, but the varying conditions and types of races demand different skills. Endurance races typically require sustained effort and tactical navigation.

The history of kayaking extends back thousands of years, with its origins rooted in the traditional watercraft of indigenous peoples, particularly those of the Arctic regions. The word "kayak" comes from the Inuit language, referring to the traditional skin-covered boats used by Arctic people for hunting and transportation. These early kayaks were crafted from materials such as wood, bone, and animal skins, designed to navigate icy waters and rough conditions. The modern sport of kayaking began to take shape in the late 19th and early 20th centuries, when the traditional designs were adapted for recreational and competitive use. The first international kayaking competition was held in Germany in 1924, and the sport gained further prominence with its inclusion in the Olympic Games in 1936. Over the years, kayaking evolved with advancements in materials and technology, such as the introduction of lightweight fiberglass and plastic kayaks, which improved performance and accessibility.

Long-distance kayaking, or marathon kayaking, has roots that can be traced back to the early 20th century, with some of the earliest endurance races held in Europe. One of the pioneering events was the "Saar Marathon" in Germany, first held in 1928, which covered a distance of 30km on the Saar River. These early marathons tested both the physical endurance and the technical skills of participants, navigating long stretches of water under varying conditions. The concept of long-distance racing gained further recognition with the establishment of the "Devizes to Westminster International Canoe Marathon" in the United Kingdom, first held in 1948.

This prestigious race covers 125 miles of river and canal, demanding extraordinary stamina and strategic planning. Early long-distance races helped to highlight the endurance capabilities required for competitive kayaking and set the stage for the development of modern marathon events.

Advances in kayak design and materials, such as carbon fibre and advanced composites, have led to lighter and more hydrodynamic vessels, allowing for faster speeds and greater manoeuvrability. Additionally, training techniques and sports science have progressed, providing kayakers with more sophisticated methods to enhance performance, endurance, and recovery. There is also now an emphasis on multi-discipline events, where kayaking is combined with other sports like running or cycling. This reflects a trend towards more complex and demanding competitions.

Several factors contribute to the difficulty of kayaking races, each adding its own set of challenges. The length and type of race are fundamental. Water conditions are a significant factor, with varying levels of turbulence, currents, and waves adding complexity to the race. The physical demands of paddling, including upper body strength and cardiovascular endurance, are amplified by factors such as wind, temperature extremes, and fatigue.

YUKON 1000

- **Location**... Canada
- **Time of year**................................. July
- **Approximate distance**................. 1600km (1000 miles)
- **Average time to finish**................. 7 – 12 days
- **Average number of entries**.......... 30 teams
- **Average cost to enter**................... $2500 – $3500
- **Year it started**............................. 2009
- **Support offered**........................... Unsupported

The Yukon 1000 is the world's longest annual kayak and canoe race, challenging participants to paddle 1000 miles across remote territories from Canada into the USA. It started in 2009, with this biennial event now testing the endurance and survival skills of its participants. It is designed for the experienced paddler looking to tackle one of the last great wilderness areas. The race promotes not only physical endurance but an unparalleled river expedition.

Navigating from Whitehorse to the Dalton Highway bridge, competitors in the Yukon 1000 face numerous challenges. The race course runs through some of North America's most isolated regions, featuring vast landscapes, wildlife, and the untouched beauty. The difficulty of the race is compounded by its length, the need for self-sufficiency, and the unpredictable elements, including variable weather conditions and river flows. Paddlers must manage their food and rest, deal with potential wildlife encounters, and maintain their equipment without any external support.

Entry into the Yukon 1000 is strictly regulated to ensure that only teams with appropriate wilderness and paddling experience participate. Teams must demonstrate extensive proof of capability, including prior experience in multi-day paddle races or equivalent wilderness expeditions. Each team must comprise at least two members for safety reasons, and all participants are required to attend a comprehensive pre-race briefing. Safety equipment, including satellite phones, GPS tracking devices, and emergency supplies, are mandatory. Teams must also adhere to strict environmental guidelines to minimize their impact on the pristine ecosystems they traverse.

You can find further details about the Yukon 1000 on their official website: https://www.yukon1000.org/

RACE TO ALASKA

- **Location**.. United States & Canada
- **Time of year**.................................... June
- **Approximate distance**................. 1207km (750 miles)
- **Average time to finish**................ 4 – 14 days
- **Average number of entries**.......... 30 teams
- **Average cost to enter**................... $500 – $800
- **Year it started**............................. 2015
- **Support offered**........................... Unsupported

The Race to Alaska, known as R2AK, is a unique, non-motorized maritime race that starts from Port Townsend, Washington, and ends in Ketchikan, Alaska. Initiated in 2015 by the Northwest Maritime Center, the race was designed to challenge the seamanship of participants in one of the most beautiful and treacherous waterways in the world. The race is open to any vessel without an engine, from rowboats to kayaks to sailboats, and has attracted a diverse array of adventurers over the years.

The R2AK offers a daunting 750 mile course through the Inside Passage, a route notorious for its tricky navigation, unpredictable weather, and strong tidal currents. The race route passes through narrow straits and remote wilderness, where encountering wildlife like whales and bears is common. The lack of any support vessels means that participants must be entirely self-reliant, capable of self-rescue, and prepared for any emergencies without expecting immediate help. The mental and physical toll, combined with the need to manage food, fatigue, and equipment, makes this race a severe test of endurance and skill.

To enter the Race to Alaska, participants must form a team (although solo entries are not unheard of) and choose a non-motorized vessel. Teams must demonstrate thorough preparation, including a survival suit for each member, and are required to attend a pre-race safety inspection to confirm that their craft is sea-worthy and properly equipped for the demanding journey. A qualifying event or proving journey must be completed in advance, such as the 40-mile "Proving Ground" from Port Townsend to Victoria, BC, to show readiness for the main event.

You can find details about the Race to Alaska on their official website:
https://r2ak.com/

MISSOURI RIVER 340

- **Location**..................................... Missouri (United States)
- **Time of year**............................... July
- **Approximate distance**................. 547km (340 miles)
- **Average time to finish**................ 40 – 88 hours
- **Average number of entries**.......... 400 – 500 boats
- **Average cost to enter**.................. $200 – $400
- **Year it started**............................. 2006
- **Support offered**........................... Semi-supported

The Missouri River 340 (MR340) is a gruelling and prestigious ultramarathon river race that began in 2006. It traverses the state of Missouri, following the Missouri River from Kansas City to St. Charles. The race was started to offer a supreme test of endurance and paddling skill while also promoting awareness of the Missouri River's ecological and historical significance. Over the years, it has grown significantly in size and popularity, attracting hundreds of paddlers to test their limits in one of the longest continuous kayak and canoe races in the world.

Participants must navigate under numerous bridges, around river bends, and through varied weather conditions, which can range from intense heat to severe thunderstorms. The challenge is heightened by the race's non-stop nature, where competitors must decide how much time to allocate paddling versus resting, often continuing through the night to gain an advantage.

Entry into the MR340 is open to various types of human-powered boats, including solo and team categories for canoes, kayaks, and stand-up paddleboards. Participants must be at least 18 years old, or 16 with parental consent. All racers are required to demonstrate their ability to swim and must attend a pre-race safety meeting. They must also provide their own support crew to meet them at designated checkpoints along the route, supplying food, water, and any necessary repairs or medical attention. Safety gear, including life jackets and navigation lights, is mandatory, which ensures participants are prepared for both daytime and nighttime conditions.

You can find details about the Missouri River 340 on their official website: https://mr340.org/

THE WATERTRIBE EVERGLADES CHALLENGE

- **Location**.. Florida (United States)
- **Time of year**.................................... March
- **Approximate distance**................. 483km (300 mile)
- **Average time to finish**................. 3 – 8 days
- **Average number of entries**.......... 100 – 150 participants
- **Average cost to enter**.................... $500
- **Year it started**............................. 2001
- **Support offered**........................... Unsupported

The WaterTribe Everglades Challenge is an annual expedition-style adventure race for small boats and kayaks that began in 2001. It is organized by WaterTribe Inc., which hosts several similar challenges designed to test the limits of participants navigation, camping, and long-distance boating. The challenge is renowned for its demands and the beautiful waters it navigates through the Florida coastline and Everglades National Park.

The course from Fort De Soto to Key Largo spans about 300 miles along the western coast of Florida, through the Ten Thousand Islands, and into the open waters of the Florida Keys. The race is particularly challenging due to the unpredictable weather, strong currents, and shallow waters that require precise navigation and strategic planning. Paddlers and sailors face physical exhaustion as they manage continuous shifts in tide and wind, navigate through mangrove swamps, and often have to portage or drag their vessels. Additionally, participants must be prepared to camp in the wild and manage all aspects of survival in remote and potentially hazardous environments.

Participants wishing to join the race must demonstrate significant self-sufficiency and a strong background in small craft handling. Entry is contingent upon passing a thorough inspection that includes safety gear, navigation equipment, and boat seaworthiness. Experience in long-distance boating and a solid understanding of coastal navigation are strongly recommended. Participants must also complete a WaterTribe training course or demonstrate equivalent experience through other maritime or adventure races.

You can find the WaterTribe Everglades Challenge on their official website:
https://www.watertribe.com/events/evergladeschallenge/

TEXAS WATER SAFARI

- **Location**.. Texas (United States)
- **Time of year**................................ June
- **Approximate distance**................. 418km (260 miles)
- **Average time to finish**................. 40 – 100 hours
- **Average number of entries**.......... 150 – 200 teams
- **Average cost to enter**.................... $200 – $400
- **Year it started**............................ 1963
- **Support offered**........................... Unsupported

The Texas Water Safari is billed as the "World's Toughest Canoe Race" and has been challenging paddlers since 1963. This annual race begins in San Marcos and ends at the Texas Gulf Coast in Seadrift. Originally started as a leisurely paddle, it quickly evolved into a competitive race. Over the decades, it has grown in fame and participation, drawing elite paddlers and adventurous spirits from across the nation and beyond, all eager to test their endurance and skill against the gruelling Texas rivers and unpredictable weather.

The 260 mile course of the Texas Water Safari passes through varied and challenging river environments, including swift-moving sections, slow stagnant waters, numerous portages, and dam bypasses. The race is made even more difficult by the scorching Texas heat, potential for severe weather, and the wildlife of the region, including alligators and snakes. Participants must be prepared to paddle both day and night, often facing sleep deprivation and extreme fatigue as they push towards the finish line.

Entry into the Texas Water Safari is open to anyone who can meet the physical and logistical demands of the race. Participants can compete in various categories, including solo and team entries. All participants must provide their own boats and paddling gear and are required to have a support team that can meet them at various checkpoints with supplies like food, water, and medical or repair kits. Prior to the race, participants must complete a series of qualifying events or prove their experience in other endurance paddle races.

You can find details about Texas Water Safari on their official website:
https://www.texaswatersafari.org/

MASSIVE MURRAY PADDLE

- **Location**... Australia
- **Time of year**................................. November
- **Approximate distance**................. 404km (251 miles)
- **Average time to finish**.................. 5 days
- **Average number of entries**.......... 350 – 400 participants
- **Average cost to enter**.................... $300 – $600
- **Year it started**.............................. 1969
- **Support offered**............................ Semi-supported

The Massive Murray Paddle, formerly known as the Murray Marathon, is an iconic Australian paddling event that has been challenging canoeists and kayakers since 1969. The race was initially established to raise funds for the YMCA and has since evolved into a celebrated sporting event that also highlights river health and supports various charities. Over the decades, it has grown in popularity and now attracts a diverse group of paddlers from across Australia and around the world, making it one of the most significant paddle races in the Southern Hemisphere.

The course covers 404km of the Murray River, passing through the Victoria-New South Wales border region. It is divided into five stages, each ranging from approximately 70 to 100km. One of the major challenges is the variability of the river itself, which can include slow-moving waters, strong currents, and various natural obstacles like snags and shallow sections. The weather can also vary significantly during the race, with potential for high temperatures and strong winds.

The Massive Murray Paddle is open to a wide range of paddlers, from experienced marathoners to enthusiastic amateurs. Participants can enter as solo paddlers or as part of a team in various boat classes, including kayaks, canoes, and outrigger canoes. All entrants must demonstrate their ability to safely manage long distances on the water, and first-time participants are encouraged to have completed some form of training or prior paddling experience to ensure they can handle the demands of the race.

You can find details about the Massive Murray Paddle on their official website: https://www.mmp415.racing/

CANOEING

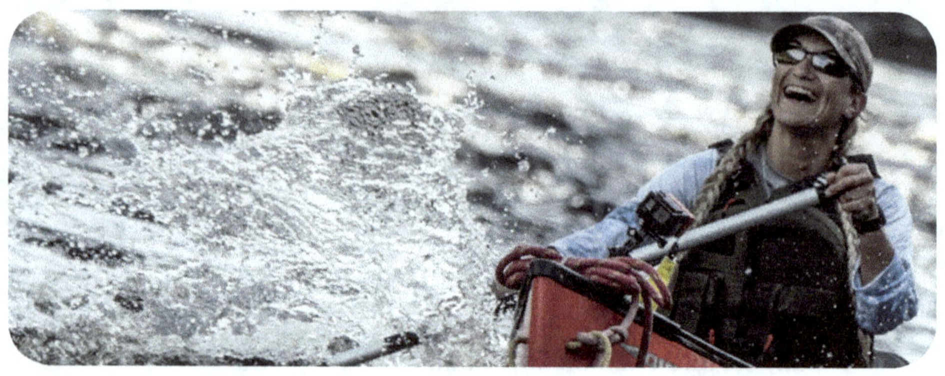

Canoeing is a competitive sport where athletes paddle a canoe or kayak to complete a designated course as quickly as possible with a single paddle. The history of canoeing is deeply intertwined with the development of early human transportation and exploration. Canoes have been used by indigenous peoples around the world for thousands of years, primarily for fishing, hunting, and travel. The earliest known canoes were constructed from hollowed-out tree trunks or crafted with bark and reeds, reflecting the ingenuity of various cultures in adapting their designs to local environments. The modern sport of canoeing began to emerge in the late 19th and early 20th centuries, as traditional canoe designs were adapted for competitive use. The International Canoe Federation (ICF) was founded in 1924, marking a formalization of the sport at the international level. Canoeing was included in the Olympic Games for the first time in 1936, showcasing its evolution from a practical means of transport to a regulated competitive sport.

The concept of long-distance canoeing races has historical roots in early endurance events that tested both the physical limits of participants. One of the earliest significant long-distance races was the "Devizes to Westminster International Canoe Marathon" in the United Kingdom, which started in 1948. Covering 125 miles, this race traverses rivers and canals, challenging athletes with its distance and varying water conditions. Another notable early event was the "Canoe Marathon World Championship," which began in the late 20th century and featured long-distance races on diverse watercourses.

Canoeing races have evolved significantly over the years, with increasing emphasis on both performance and the challenge of varying conditions. Advances in canoe design, including the use of high-tech materials like carbon fiber and Kevlar, have made boats lighter and faster, enabling athletes to push the boundaries of speed and efficiency. Training techniques have also become more sophisticated, incorporating sports science, nutrition, and biomechanics to enhance performance and endurance.

Additionally, technological innovations like GPS tracking and advanced water monitoring systems provide more precise data for race strategy and safety.

Several factors contribute to the difficulty of canoeing races, each presenting its own set of challenges. The distance of the race is a primary factor, with longer races requiring sustained endurance. Water conditions significantly impact the difficulty; calm, flat water allows for more straightforward navigation, while rough or turbulent water requires greater skill and adaptability. Environmental factors such as weather conditions, water temperature, and currents also play a crucial role, influencing performance and safety. Additionally, in team races, coordination and communication among crew members add a layer of complexity. Together, these elements combine to make canoeing races a multifaceted and challenging sport that tests a wide range of physical and mental skills.

LA RUTA MAYA BELIZE RIVER CHALLENGE

- **Location**..................................... Belize
- **Time of year**.............................. March
- **Approximate distance**................. 290km (180 miles)
- **Average time to finish**................ 4 days
- **Average number of entries**.......... 100 teams
- **Average cost to enter**.................. $200 – $400
- **Year it started**............................ 1998
- **Support offered**.......................... Supported

The La Ruta Maya Belize River Challenge is one of Belize's premier sporting events, drawing competitors from around the world. Established in 1998, the race was initially conceived as a way to raise awareness of environmental issues along the Belize River and promote the preservation of an important part of the country. It has now grown into a significant annual event that combines intense physical challenge with a celebration of Belizean culture and history, attracting a diverse mix of local and international teams.

The course covers 180miles of the Belize River, presenting a test of endurance, teamwork, and river navigation skills. Participants face numerous natural challenges, including strong currents, rapids, along with the logistical challenges of managing food, rest, and equipment over four continuous days of competition. The tropical climate of Belize adds another layer of difficulty, with high temperatures and humidity testing the stamina and resilience of even the most experienced paddlers. Wildlife sightings along the river, such as crocodiles and various bird species, add to the adventure of the race.

To participate in the La Ruta Maya Belize River Challenge, teams must register in one of several categories, including Professional, Amateur, Mixed, Masters, Family Adventure, and Intramural. Each team typically consists of up to four paddlers. Entrants must demonstrate a good level of physical fitness and should ideally have some experience in canoeing or kayaking, particularly in long-distance events. Teams are responsible for their own boats, which must meet the safety requirements stipulated by the organizers.

You can find details about La Ruta Maya Belize Challenge on their website: https://larutamaya.bz/

DEVIZES TO WESTMINSTER INTERNATIONAL CANOE RACE (DW)

- **Location**.. United Kingdom
- **Time of year**................................. April
- **Approximate distance**................. 200km (125 miles)
- **Average time to finish**................. 20 – 30 hours
- **Average number of entries**.......... 200 – 300 participants
- **Average cost to enter**................... $80 – $150
- **Year it started**............................. 1948
- **Support offered**........................... Supported

The DW canoe race is one of the most challenging and prestigious endurance canoe and kayak races in the world. Established in 1948, the race traces its origins to the post-World War II era when it was conceived to provide a rigorous test for canoeists and promote the sport. The event is renowned for its demanding nature and is often described as the "Kona of Canoeing" due to its difficulty and significance in the paddling community. The race spans 125 miles from Devizes in Wiltshire to Westminster in London, following a mix of canals and river sections. It has become a hallmark of endurance paddling, drawing elite athletes and enthusiasts from across the globe.

The race navigates a diverse range of water conditions, including the Kennet and Avon Canal, which presents a combination of narrow, winding stretches and technical sections. They then transition onto the Thames River, where they encounter swift currents and potential obstacles such as locks and weirs. The course includes several portages, where paddlers must carry their boats overland around locks and other obstructions, adding a significant physical and logistical challenge. The race often spans up to 24 hours, requiring participants to paddle through day and night, dealing with fatigue, changing weather conditions, and varying water levels.

To enter the race, competitors are typically required to have experience in long-distance paddling and must demonstrate their capability to complete the race within the allotted time, which is generally up to 24 hours for solo paddlers and 28 hours for teams.

You can find further information about DW Canoe race on their official website: https://www.dwrace.co.uk/

AUSABLE RIVER CANOE MARATHON

- **Location**.................................... Michigan (United States)
- **Time of year**............................... July
- **Approximate distance**................ 193km (120 miles)
- **Average time to finish**................ 14 – 19 hours
- **Average number of entries**.......... 100 teams
- **Average cost to enter**................... $300 – $400
- **Year it started**............................. 1947
- **Support offered**........................... Supported

The AuSable River Canoe Marathon is one of the longest and most prestigious canoe races in North America. Starting in 1947, it has become a highlight of the summer season in Michigan, drawing competitors and spectators from across the United States and Canada. Part of the Triple Crown of Canoe Racing, this overnight race tests paddlers' endurance, skill, and teamwork under the stars of northern Michigan.

Starting at night in Grayling, the AuSable River Canoe Marathon plunges participants into darkness as they navigate the winding, tree-lined AuSable River. The race continues non-stop through the night and into the next day, challenging teams with narrow river sections, swift currents, and numerous portages around dams and shallow areas. One of the most physically demanding parts of the race are the portages, where racers must carry their canoes on land, while still racing against the clock. The combination of nocturnal navigation, physical exhaustion from continuous paddling make this marathon a formidable challenge.

Entry requires competitors to demonstrate proficiency in canoe handling, which can be evidenced by participation in other canoe races or by completing a qualification race earlier in the year in Grayling. Teams consist of two paddlers, and both members must be prepared for the physicality of non-stop paddling and portaging. Safety gear, including life jackets and navigation lights, is mandatory, and all participants must attend pre-race meetings to review rules, safety protocols, and course details.

You can find the AuSable River Canoe Marathon on their official website:
https://www.ausablecanoemarathon.org/

ADIRONDACK CANOE CLASSIC

- **Location**.................................... New York (United States)
- **Time of year**................................ September
- **Approximate distance**.................. 145km (90 miles)
- **Average time to finish**................. 3 days
- **Average number of entries**.......... 300 participants
- **Average cost to enter**................... $150 – $275
- **Year it started**............................. 1983
- **Support offered**............................ Supported

The Adirondack Canoe Classic, also known as the "90-Miler," is a premier canoe and kayak race that traverses the Adirondack Park in New York. It draws a diverse group of paddlers, from competitive racers to recreational enthusiasts, who come to experience the Adrondack waterways.

The 90-mile course is divided into three legs, each completed over one day, making it both a test of endurance and strategic paddling. The route includes a mix of large open water bodies and narrow, winding river sections, requiring adept handling and navigation skills. Additionally, several portages where participants must carry their boats over land add to the physical challenge. The unpredictable mountain weather can also turn the waters choppy, presenting further difficulties. The combination of long distances, varied water conditions, and the necessity of portaging makes this race a demanding endeavour even for seasoned paddlers.

Participants looking to enter the Adirondack Canoe Classic must be prepared for the physical demands of a long-distance paddling event. The race is open to various types of canoes, kayaks, and guide boats. Entry categories accommodate solo paddlers, tandems, and teams. All participants are required to demonstrate adequate preparation for the race, including having the necessary equipment such as life vests, bailing devices, and whistles. While some race experience is beneficial, there are no strict prerequisites beyond the ability to manage potentially strenuous paddling and portaging. Registrants must also comply with the environmental and safety regulations set forth by the organizers to ensure a safe and responsible event.

You can find details about Adirondack Canoe Classic on their official website: https://www.northernforestcanoetrail.org/adirondack90miler/

DUSI CANOE MARATHON

- **Location**..................................... South Africa
- **Time of year**............................... February
- **Approximate distance**................. 120km (75 miles)
- **Average time to finish**................. 10 – 15 hours
- **Average number of entries**.......... 1000 participants
- **Average cost to enter**.................. $50 – $100
- **Year it started**............................ 1951
- **Support offered**........................... Supported

The Dusi Canoe Marathon is one of the most iconic canoe marathons in the world, held annually in South Africa's KwaZulu-Natal province. Established in 1951 by Dr. Ian Player, the race was originally a personal challenge to navigate the rivers between Pietermaritzburg and Durban. Over the decades, it has grown into a major sporting event, attracting elite paddlers and adventure enthusiasts from around the globe. The race is renowned for its combination of paddling and portaging, where competitors must carry their boats overland around obstacles and rapids, which adds to the already demanding course.

The Dusi Canoe Marathon course spans approximately 120km, winding through the Valley of a Thousand Hills, from the Umsindusi River in Pietermaritzburg to the Umgeni River in Durban. The race is divided into three stages over three days, each offering its own set of challenges. Competitors must navigate a mix of fast-flowing river sections, technical rapids, and long flat-water stretches. One of the unique aspects of the Dusi is the requirement to portage around dangerous rapids and shallow sections of the river. This involves carrying the canoe overland, sometimes for several kilometres, often over steep and rugged terrain. The combination of paddling, portaging, and the physical demands of the race, coupled with the heat and humidity of the South African summer, make the Dusi one of the most difficult canoe marathons in the world.

Entry is open to paddlers of all levels, but it is not for the faint-hearted. While there are no strict qualification requirements, participants are strongly encouraged to have significant experience in river paddling and to be in excellent physical condition. The Dusi Canoe Marathon is not just a race but a rite of passage for South African paddlers.

 You can find details about the Dusi Canoe Marathon on their official website: https://dusi.co.za/

THE HAWKESBURY CANOE CLASSIC

- **Location**............................... Australia
- **Time of year**............................ October
- **Approximate distance**................ 111km (69 miles)
- **Average time to finish**................ 8 – 15 hours
- **Average number of entries**.......... 600 – 800 participants
- **Average cost to enter**.................. $100 – $200
- **Year it started**........................... 1977
- **Support offered**........................ Supported

The Hawkesbury Canoe Classic is a celebrated annual paddling event that challenges kayakers and canoeists to navigate 111km of the Hawkesbury River by moonlight. Established in 1977, this overnight marathon was initially organised to support the Arrow Bone Marrow Transplant Foundation, and it has continued to raise funds for medical research and patient support. The event has become a fixture in the Australian paddling community, known for its challenging nature and its festive atmosphere.

Starting in Windsor and finishing in Brooklyn, the course follows the winding Hawkesbury River. Paddling overnight adds a significant layer of difficulty to the race, as visibility is reduced, and paddlers must rely on their lights and navigational skills to safely manoeuvre through the river's bends and currents.

To participate in the Hawkesbury Canoe Classic, paddlers must demonstrate a level of fitness and experience appropriate for an overnight long-distance event. Both solo paddlers and teams can enter, with various boat classes allowed, including kayaks, canoes, and outrigger canoes. All entrants are required to have a support crew to meet them at designated checkpoints to provide logistical and moral support. Safety is paramount, so mandatory gear includes life jackets, adequate lighting, and a whistle. Participants must also attend a pre-race safety briefing to ensure they are fully prepared for the conditions of the night race.

You can find info about the Hawkesbury Canoe Classic on their official website: https://www.canoeclassic.net/enter

SAILING

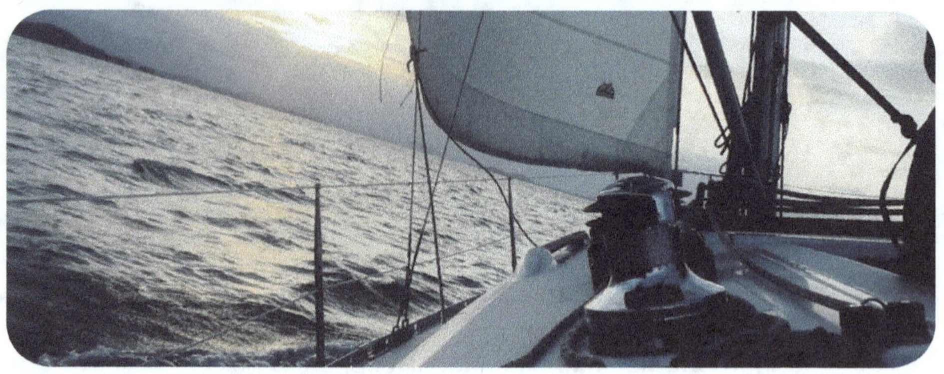

Sailing, in the context of racing, is a competitive sport where participants manoeuvre boats using the wind's power to navigate a designated course as quickly as possible. Racing formats vary widely, from short, tactical races in confined waters to long, challenging ocean voyages. Offshore racing covers long distances and can involve navigating through challenging sea conditions. Different types of boats are used in racing, including dinghies, catamarans, and larger yachts, each with its own set of rules and strategies. Key elements of sailing races include sail trim, boat handling, wind shifts, and strategic positioning relative to competitors.

The history of sailing as a competitive sport dates back to ancient times, where it was first practiced by early civilizations such as the Egyptians, Greeks, and Romans for trade, exploration, and warfare. The concept of racing under sail likely evolved from these early uses, with evidence of competitive sailing appearing in the medieval period. By the 17th century, organized sailing races began to take shape in Europe, particularly in England, where the Royal Yacht Squadron was established in 1815. The sport's formalization continued with the creation of the America's Cup in 1851, the world's oldest international sporting trophy, which marked a significant milestone in competitive sailing. The 20th century saw further development with the inclusion of sailing in the Olympic Games starting in 1900.

The early long-endurance sailing races have their roots in the 19th century, when sailors began to push the limits of long-distance ocean voyages in competitive formats. One of the earliest notable endurance races was the transatlantic race, exemplified by the first transatlantic sailing race held in 1866, from New York to London. This race highlighted the challenges of long-distance sailing and tested the limits of navigation and endurance over vast oceanic distances. The first modern solo non-stop transatlantic race was undertaken by Sir Francis Chichester in 1960, who completed the voyage in 120 days, setting a benchmark for future endurance events. These early long-distance races underscored the extreme demands placed on sailors.

Sailing races have become increasingly demanding and sophisticated, reflecting advancements in technology and evolving competitive standards. The evolution of boat design has been a major factor in this progression, with innovations in materials and construction techniques leading to faster and more agile vessels. Modern racing yachts often feature advanced aerodynamic and hydrodynamic designs, such as foiling technology, which allows boats to lift out of the water and achieve higher speeds. Training techniques and tactical strategies have also advanced, with sailors using sophisticated weather forecasting tools, GPS tracking, and performance analytics to gain a competitive edge. The rise of high-profile races such as the Volvo Ocean Race and the Vendée Globe, which involve circumnavigating the globe solo or in teams, highlights the increasing complexity and endurance required in modern sailing.

The difficulty of a sailing race is influenced by multiple factors, each contributing to the overall challenge of the event. The complexity of sailing races comes from the interplay of wind conditions, sea state, and navigation. Sailors must constantly adjust their sails and boat trim to respond to changing wind speeds and directions, requiring a high degree of skill and adaptability. In offshore races, the challenge is compounded by long distances, unpredictable weather, and the need for self-sufficiency, as sailors must manage their resources and maintain their vessel over extended periods. The physical demands of sailing include managing heavy sails, enduring harsh weather conditions, and handling the physical stress of long hours at sea.

VOLVO OCEAN RACE

- **Location**...................................... World
- **Time of year**................................ October (every three years)
- **Approximate distance**................. 83,340km(45,000 nautical miles)
- **Average time to finish**................ 8 – 9 months
- **Average number of entries**.......... 7 – 11 teams
- **Average cost to enter**.................. $1,000,000
- **Year it started**............................ 1973
- **Support offered**........................... Semi-supported

The Volvo Ocean Race is known as the world's premier offshore sailing competition. It began in 1973 as the Whitbread Round the World Race and has grown in prestige and complexity to become a highlight in the international sailing calendar, attracting top sailors and major sponsors. The race spans multiple legs across the world's most challenging oceans. It was rebranded in 2001 when Volvo took over the title sponsorship, and it has continued to evolve with advancements in boat technology and race logistics.

The course is designed to be one of the most demanding in sailing, often requiring teams to navigate through treacherous conditions such as the icy waters of the Southern Ocean, the notorious Cape Horn, and the tricky weather systems of the North and South Atlantic. The race tests the crews abilities to cope with extreme fatigue, harsh weather, and constant tactical decision-making. The use of one design racing yachts in recent editions has heightened the competition, focusing more on team skills and strategy rather than technological advantages.

Entry into the race is a lengthy process, requiring significant commitment from teams and their sponsors. Competitors are often professional sailors with vast experience in ocean racing. Teams must secure substantial funding to cover the design and construction of a competitive yacht, training, team salaries, and race logistics. Each team must comply with strict safety and training standards set by the race organizers, including completion of qualification sails and participation in pre-race safety courses. The race emphasizes sustainability and innovation, with recent editions focusing on reducing environmental impact and promoting ocean health awareness.

You can find details about the Volvo Ocean Race on their official website: https://www.theoceanrace.com/

CLIPPER ROUND THE WORLD YACHT RACE

- **Location**.. World
- **Time of year**.................................... August (every two years)
- **Approximate distance**.................. 874,000km(40,000 nautical miles)
- **Average time to finish**.................. 11 months
- **Average number of entries**.......... 12 teams
- **Average cost to enter**................... $5000 – $50,000
- **Year it started**.............................. 1996
- **Support offered**............................ Supported

The Clipper Round the World Yacht Race is a unique event designed to give amateur sailors the chance to experience the challenges of round-the-world ocean racing. Founded in 1996 by Sir Robin Knox-Johnston, the first person to sail solo non-stop around the world, the Clipper Race aims to make ocean racing accessible to people from various walks of life without prior sailing experience. The race has grown significantly in scope and popularity since its beginning, attracting a diverse group of participants and global sponsorship.

The Clipper Race circumnavigates the globe, starting and finishing in the UK, with the route divided into a series of legs that stop at ports across continents. The race features some of the world's most challenging seas, including the notorious Southern Ocean, the North Pacific, and the complex weather systems of the South Atlantic. Participants face enormous physical and mental challenges, dealing with extreme weather conditions, high seas, and the complexities of long-distance team sailing.

To join the Clipper Race, no previous sailing experience is required, which sets it apart from other global yacht races. Participants must be over 18 and pass a rigorous training program provided by the Clipper Race organization, designed to equip them with the necessary skills to safely navigate a yacht under racing conditions. This training includes sea survival, sail handling, navigation, and race tactics. Participants can choose to race one leg, several legs, or the entire circumnavigation. Each crew member is required to demonstrate not only physical fitness but also the psychological resilience needed to cope with the extreme demands of ocean racing.

You can find details about the Clipper Round The World Race on their website: https://www.clipperroundtheworld.com/

GOLDEN GLOBE RACE

- **Location**....................................... World
- **Time of year**............................... September
- **Approximate distance**................. 55,560km (30,000 nautical miles)
- **Average time to finish**................ 240 – 300 days
- **Average number of entries**.......... 20 – 25 boats
- **Average cost to enter**.................. $10,000 – $15,000
- **Year it started**............................. 1968
- **Support offered**........................... Unsupported

The Golden Globe Race is one of the most challenging and storied solo sailing competitions in the world. The race was conceived by the Sunday Times to celebrate the first single-handed circumnavigation of the globe. The original race, won by Sir Robin Knox-Johnston, remains a landmark in sailing history, as he became the first person to sail solo and non-stop around the world. The race was revived in 2018 to commemorate the 50th anniversary of the original event, adhering to the same traditional rules.

The race course starts and finishes in Les Sables-d'Olonne, France. The route takes competitors down the Atlantic Ocean, around the Cape of Good Hope, across the Southern Ocean beneath the continents of Africa, Australia, and South America, and then back up the Atlantic to France. The race route follows the "Clipper Route," known for its harsh weather, massive swells, and the notorious Southern Ocean, where sailors face the Roaring Forties, Furious Fifties, and Shrieking Sixties, which are latitudes infamous for their relentless winds and towering waves. The difficulty of the race is compounded by the fact that competitors are restricted to using technology available in 1968, meaning no GPS, autopilots, or electronic aids are allowed. Sailors must rely on celestial navigation, sextants, and paper charts, making navigation and weather prediction extremely challenging. The isolation, physical exhaustion, and mental strain of being alone at sea for up to 10 months make the Golden Globe Race one of the toughest endurance events in the world.

Prospective entrants must have experience in solo ocean sailing, including at least 8,000 nautical miles of ocean sailing, with a minimum of 2,000 miles solo. They must also complete a qualifying sail of 2,000 miles in their chosen boat. The boats themselves must be production boats designed before 1988, between 32 and 36 feet in length, and built to specific safety standards.

You can find details about the Golden Globe race on their official website: https://goldengloberace.com/

VENDEE GLOBE

- **Location**.. World
- **Time of year**................................. November (every four years)
- **Approximate distance**.................. 44,450km(24,000 nautical miles)
- **Average time to finish**................. 70 – 100 days
- **Average number of entries**.......... 20 – 30 teams
- **Average cost to enter**................... $1,000,000
- **Year it started**.............................. 1989
- **Support offered**........................... Unsupported

The Vendée Globe is the pinnacle of single-handed offshore racing, famously known as the "Everest of the Seas." Initiated in 1989 by Philippe Jeantot, the race takes place every four years and has grown in prominence within the sailing world. It is unique as it requires skippers to race non-stop around the world, without assistance, making it one of the most gruelling physical and mental challenges in sport. The race starts and finishes in Les Sables-d'Olonne, France, and has seen many dramatic moments and technological advancements over the decades.

The course involves circumnavigating the globe from the Atlantic Ocean into the Indian Ocean, rounding Cape of Good Hope, passing Australia's Cape Leeuwin, and rounding Cape Horn back into the Atlantic. The route tests skippers against some of the most extreme weather conditions on earth, particularly in the Southern Ocean, known for monstrous waves and fierce winds. The solitude of the race, combined with the relentless need to manage the boat's technology and perform all necessary repairs while navigating, makes this race extraordinarily challenging.

Entry requires significant offshore racing experience, particularly in the IMOCA 60 class, which is the boat class used for the race. Skippers must qualify by completing specific races and accumulating sufficient miles at sea under racing conditions. They must also manage a substantial campaign, securing funding for boat construction or refurbishment, technology, training, and logistics. Safety is paramount, and all entrants must undergo rigorous safety training, including survival at sea courses.

You can find details about Vendee Globe on their official website:
https://www.vendeeglobe.org/en

TRANSAT JACQUES VABRE

- **Location**.. France to Brazil
- **Time of year**.................................. October
- **Approximate distance**.................. 8056km (4,350 nautical miles)
- **Average time to finish**.................. 10 – 16 days
- **Average number of entries**.......... 60 – 80 boats
- **Average cost to enter**.................... $1500 – $3000
- **Year it started**.............................. 1993
- **Support offered**............................ Semi-supported

The Transat Jacques Vabre is one of the most prestigious transatlantic yacht races, held biennially since 1993. Named after the French coffee brand Jacques Vabre, the race was initially conceived to celebrate the historic coffee trade route between France and South America. The race is unique as it is a double-handed (two-person) race, requiring exceptional teamwork and skill. Over the years, it has grown in prominence, attracting some of the world's best sailors and becoming a key event in the sailing calendar. The race has evolved in terms of its destination, initially ending in Cartagena, Colombia, before moving to Salvador de Bahia, Brazil, and more recently to Martinique in the Caribbean.

Competitors must navigate through the English Channel, the Bay of Biscay, and the trade winds of the Atlantic, which can present anything from light breezes to powerful gales. The race also involves crossing the notorious Doldrums near the equator, where calm winds and squalls can trap boats for days. The diversity of the fleet, which includes IMOCA 60s, Class40s, and Ocean Fifty multihulls, means that strategies vary widely depending on the type of boat and its strengths. The double-handed format adds an extra layer of difficulty, as the two sailors must manage all aspects of the race themselves, including navigation, sail changes, and repairs, while also finding time to rest.

Entry requires sailors to prove their capability in offshore racing, typically through participation in qualifying races or other major offshore events. Teams must also ensure their boats are in peak condition to handle the rigors of the transatlantic crossing.

You can find details about the Transat Jacques Vabre on their official website:
https://www.transatjacquesvabre.org/en

TRANSATLANTIC RACE

- **Location**.................................... United States &
  United Kingdom
- **Time of year**............................... June
- **Approximate distance**................. 5185km (3000 nautical miles)
- **Average time to finish**................. 10 – 20 days
- **Average number of entries**.......... 30 – 40 boats
- **Average cost to enter**................... $2500 – $5000
- **Year it started**.............................. 1866
- **Support offered**........................... Semi-supported

The Transatlantic Race is one of the oldest ocean races in the world, with a history dating back to 1866 when the first transatlantic yacht race was held between three schooners. The race has evolved significantly since its inception, with the modern iteration being re-established in 2011 under the joint organization of the Royal Yacht Squadron, New York Yacht Club, Royal Ocean Racing Club, and Storm Trysail Club. This race takes sailors from Newport, Rhode Island, across the North Atlantic to Cowes on the Isle of Wight, UK. The Transatlantic Race is held every four years and attracts some of the world's top offshore sailors, along with a diverse fleet of yachts, ranging from classic vessels to state-of-the-art racing machines.

Competitors face a myriad of challenges, including strong currents, variable winds, and the potential for severe weather systems, such as low-pressure systems that can bring gale-force winds and large ocean swells. The route also crosses the cold Labrador Current, which can cause fog and unpredictable weather conditions. The sheer length of the race requires meticulous planning, with navigators needing to make strategic decisions about routing and sail selection, often days in advance.

Entry requires boats to be offshore-capable and meet specific safety standards, including the completion of a comprehensive safety inspection before the race.

You can find details about Transatlantic Race on their official website: https://rorctransatlantic.rorc.org/

TRANSPACIFIC YACHT RACE

- **Location**.. United States
- **Time of year**................................ July
- **Approximate distance**................. 4121km (2225 nautical miles)
- **Average time to finish**................ 8 – 14 days
- **Average number of entries**.......... 50 – 70 boats
- **Average cost to enter**................... $1500 – $4000
- **Year it started**............................. 1906
- **Support offered**............................ Semi-supported

The Transpacific Yacht Race, commonly known as the Transpac was first held in 1906, the race was established by Hawaii's King Kalākaua to strengthen ties between Hawaii and the mainland United States through the sport of sailing. The race takes competitors from the mainland port of Los Angeles, California, across the Pacific Ocean to Honolulu, Hawaii. The Transpac has become an iconic event in the sailing community, known for its combination of challenging ocean conditions, the allure of the Pacific trade winds, and the warm Hawaiian welcome that awaits the finishers.

Competitors must navigate the vast expanse of the Pacific Ocean, which presents a unique set of challenges. The early part of the race often involves light and variable winds, requiring careful navigation and strategic sail handling. As the fleet moves farther offshore, they typically encounter the strong trade winds that drive the fast and exhilarating downwind sailing for which the Transpac is famous. However, the Pacific Ocean can also be unpredictable, with the potential for squalls, high seas, and the occasional calm patches that test the patience and skill of the crew.

Entry into the Transpac is open to experienced offshore sailors and boats that meet the rigorous safety and technical standards set by the race organizers, the Transpacific Yacht Club. All participating yachts must undergo a comprehensive safety inspection before the race, ensuring they are equipped with the necessary safety gear. The skipper and a percentage of the crew must have completed a qualifying offshore race and must attend a certified safety and sea survival course.

You can find further details about Transpac race on their official website:
https://transpacyc.com/

ROLEX FASTNET RACE

- **Location**... United Kingdom
- **Time of year**................................. July
- **Approximate distance**................. 1287km (695 nautical miles)
- **Average time to finish**................ 4 – 5 days
- **Average number of entries**.......... 300 boats
- **Average cost to enter**................... $1250 – $2500
- **Year it started**............................ 1925
- **Support offered**.......................... Semi-supported

The Rolex Fastnet Race, first held in 1925, is one of the world's most renowned offshore yacht races. Organized by the Royal Ocean Racing Club, the race takes competitors from Cowes, on the Isle of Wight, around the iconic Fastnet Rock off the southern coast of Ireland, before finishing in Plymouth, UK. Known for its combination of challenging weather conditions and the strategic demands of navigating varied coastal and offshore waters, the Fastnet Race has become a symbol of endurance and skill in the global sailing community.

The Rolex Fastnet Race is notorious for its unpredictable and often treacherous conditions. Competitors face the complexities of coastal navigation along the English Channel before venturing into the open waters of the Celtic Sea. Fast-changing weather, strong tides, and the potential for storms add to the challenge. Rounding Fastnet Rock, a key milestone in the race, offers both a tactical turning point and a dramatic moment of relief for sailors before they head back toward Plymouth. The race is a true test of seamanship, as crews must balance endurance with strategy over the approximately 695 nautical mile course.

Entry into the Fastnet Race is open to experienced sailors with boats that meet strict safety standards set by the Royal Ocean Racing Club. All participating yachts undergo rigorous safety inspections, and skippers, along with a portion of their crew, are required to complete qualifying offshore races prior to participation. Additionally, crews must attend safety training courses, ensuring that they are well-prepared for the demanding conditions that this iconic race presents.

You can find details about the Rolex Fastnet Race on their official website:
https://www.rolexfastnetrace.com/en

BERMUDA RACE

- **Location**.. United States & Bermuda
- **Time of year**.................................. June
- **Approximate distance**.................. 1176km (635 nautical miles)
- **Average time to finish**.................. 2 – 6 days
- **Average number of entries**.......... 150 – 200 boats
- **Average cost to enter**................... $1500 – $3500
- **Year it started**............................. 1906
- **Support offered**........................... Semi-supported

The Bermuda race, first held in 1906, the race was founded by Thomas Fleming Day, a yachting writer and avid sailor who believed in the importance of safety and seamanship in ocean racing. Over the decades, the Bermuda Race has grown into a cornerstone event in the sailing world, attracting top sailors and yachts from around the globe. The race is held biennially, beginning in Newport, Rhode Island, and ending in the tropical waters of Bermuda.

While the race distance might seem manageable, the race is notorious for its challenging conditions. Sailors must navigate the Gulf Stream, a powerful ocean current that can present significant navigational challenges and unpredictable weather. The Gulf Stream's strong currents and eddies can lead to rapid changes in wind and sea state, making the race as much about strategy as it is about speed. Competitors must also be prepared for the potential of encountering severe storms, heavy fog, and the ever-present risk of equipment failure far from shore.

Entry into the Bermuda Race is open to sailors and yachts that meet stringent qualifications, reflecting the race's emphasis on safety and preparedness. Boats must be offshore-capable and meet specific safety standards, including safety inspections before the race. Skippers and crews are required to have experience in offshore racing, and a certain percentage of the crew must have completed a safety at sea seminar within the last five years.

You can find details about Bermuda Race on their official website:
https://bermudarace.com/

SYDNEY TO HOBART YACHT RACE

- **Location**... Australia
- **Time of year**............................... December
- **Approximate distance**................. 1166km (628 nautical miles)
- **Average time to finish**................. 2 – 4 days
- **Average number of entries**.......... 100 boats
- **Average cost to enter**................... $2500 – $6000
- **Year it started**............................. 1945
- **Support offered**........................... Semi-supported

The Sydney to Hobart Yacht Race is one of the most iconic ocean races in the world, held annually since 1945. The race starts on Boxing Day (December 26) in Sydney Harbour and finishes in Hobart, the capital of Tasmania. Organized by the Cruising Yacht Club of Australia (CYCA), the race has grown from a local event into an international sporting spectacle that attracts elite sailors and yachts from around the globe. The race is a key fixture in the Australian summer sporting calendar and draws significant media attention, with the start in Sydney Harbour being a major event watched by thousands.

The course of the Sydney to Hobart Yacht Race spans 628 nautical miles, taking competitors from the bustling waters of Sydney Harbour, down the south-eastern coast of Australia, across the Bass Strait, and into the often treacherous waters of the Tasman Sea before reaching the Derwent River and the finish line in Hobart. The race is notorious for the challenging conditions it can present, particularly in the Bass Strait, where the shallow waters can create steep, breaking waves, and in the Tasman Sea, where yachts can encounter strong winds and large swells.

Entry into the Sydney to Hobart Yacht Race is open to offshore-capable yachts that meet the strict safety and technical standards set by the CYCA. All participating yachts must pass a comprehensive safety inspection before the race, ensuring they are equipped with the necessary safety gear. Skippers and a percentage of the crew must have completed a qualifying offshore race and must undergo a certified safety and sea survival course.

You can find details about the Sydney to Hobart race on their official website: https://rolexsydneyhobart.com/

STAND-UP PADDLEBOARDING

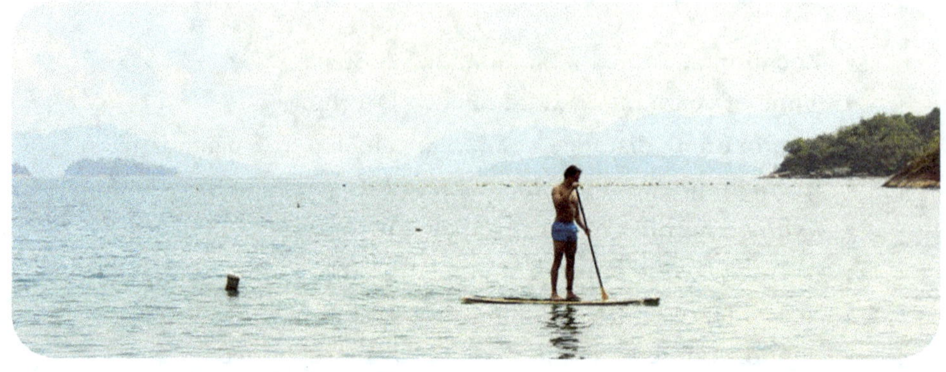

Stand up paddleboarding (SUP) racing is a dynamic sport where participants use a paddle to propel themselves while standing on a board. This relatively modern water sport can be categorized into several race formats, each presenting unique challenges and requiring different skill sets. SUP races can be held in diverse conditions, such as river currents, ocean swells, or choppy lakes, further testing participants' adaptability and endurance. The sport requires a blend of balance, strength, and technique, making it both physically demanding and strategically complex.

Stand up paddleboarding has roots that trace back to ancient cultures, but its modern iteration began to take shape in the mid-20th century. Early forms of paddleboarding can be seen in traditional Polynesian cultures, where ancient Hawaiians used similar techniques for transportation and fishing. The modern revival of SUP is credited to the surf culture of the 1960s in Hawaii. During this period, surfers started standing on their boards and using paddles to take photos or keep an eye on the waves, which evolved into a new form of water sport. This practice became more formalized in the early 2000s when SUP boards and paddles were commercially produced, leading to the sport's growth in popularity worldwide. The International Stand Up Paddleboarding Association (ISUPA) and other governing bodies began to organize competitions and establish rules, further formalizing the sport. By the mid-2000s, SUP racing had gained significant traction, with events ranging from local races to international championships. The sport's rapid growth reflects its accessibility, versatility, and appeal across different water environments.

The concept of long-distance stand up paddleboarding races began to gain prominence as the sport evolved from its recreational roots into a competitive discipline. One of the earliest notable long-distance SUP races was the "Molokai 2 Oahu Paddleboard Race," which has been held annually since 1997. This race, which covers approximately 32 miles across the channel between the Hawaiian islands of Molokai and Oahu, is one of the most challenging endurance events in the sport. It tests participants' stamina, navigation skills, and ability to handle ocean swells and changing weather conditions.

Another significant early endurance race is the "Battle of the Paddle," which started in 2008 and quickly became a premier event in the SUP racing calendar, featuring both long-distance and technical races. These pioneering endurance races set a high bar for the sport, demonstrating the physical and mental challenges of long-distance paddling and establishing benchmarks for future events.

The evolution of SUP racing has led to increasingly demanding and sophisticated competitions, driven by advancements in equipment, training, and race formats. Modern SUP boards have seen significant technological improvements, with innovations in materials and design enhancing speed, stability, and manoeuvrability. The development of lightweight, high-performance boards and ergonomic paddles has allowed athletes to push the boundaries of speed and endurance. Training methods have also advanced, incorporating specialized conditioning, technique refinement, and data-driven performance analysis. The variety of race formats has expanded, including ultra-endurance races, multi-day events, and challenging courses with natural obstacles such as river rapids and ocean waves.

Several factors contribute to the difficulty of stand up paddleboarding races, each adding layers of complexity to the challenge. The distance of the race plays a crucial role, longer races demand sustained endurance, effective pacing, and the ability to manage fatigue over time. Water conditions are another significant factor; competitors must navigate varying environments such as choppy waters, strong currents, and ocean swells, which test their adaptability and paddling skills. In technical races, the need to execute precise turns and manoeuvres around buoys or obstacles adds a further challenge. The physical demands of the sport include upper body strength, core stability, and cardiovascular endurance, all of which are essential for maintaining speed and balance.

YUKON RIVER QUEST

- **Location**..................................... Yukon (Canada)
- **Time of year**.............................. June
- **Approximate distance**................. 715km (444 miles)
- **Average time to finish**................ 50 – 60 hours
- **Average number of entries**.......... 100
- **Average cost to enter**.................. $750 – $1,200
- **Year it started**............................ 1999
- **Support offered**........................... Semi-supported

The Yukon River Quest, known as "the race to the midnight sun," is one of the world's longest annual marathon paddling races. It began in 1999, growing out of the excitement and heritage of river travel in the Yukon during the Klondike Gold Rush era. This race attracts paddlers from all over the globe who come to challenge themselves against the demanding conditions of the Yukon River.

The Yukon River Quest tests paddlers with a course that runs from Whitehorse to Dawson City, navigating the winding waters of the Yukon River. The race is conducted under continuous daylight, a unique aspect that aligns with the summer solstice, allowing for nearly 24-hour daylight navigation. Paddlers face numerous challenges, including cold water temperatures, variable weather conditions, and the potential for wildlife encounters. Additionally, the psychological strain of long hours of non-stop paddling, coupled with minimal sleep during the mandatory rest periods, adds to the race's difficulty. The river's remote nature also means that while there are safety boats and checkpoints, teams must be prepared for self-rescue and long periods without external support.

Participants in the Yukon River Quest must demonstrate a high level of physical fitness and paddling proficiency. While previous experience in marathon paddling is not mandatory, it is highly recommended. All participants must complete a comprehensive registration process that includes providing details on their paddling experience, equipment, and emergency preparedness. Safety gear, such as life jackets, dry suits or wetsuits, and emergency communication devices, is mandatory.

You can find details about Yukon River Quest on their official website:
https://www.yukonriverquest.com/

SUP 11 CITY TOUR

- **Location**.. Netherlands
- **Time of year**.................................... September
- **Approximate distance**.................. 220km (137 miles)
- **Average time to finish**.................. 5 days
- **Average number of entries**.......... 200 participants
- **Average cost to enter**.................... $500
- **Year it started**.............................. 2009
- **Support offered**............................ Supported

The SUP 11-City Tour, originally designed for stand-up paddleboarders, has expanded to include kayak categories, recognising the growing interest in endurance kayaking. The event takes inspiration from a historic ice-skating tour, which is held when the canals in Friesland freeze over. The kayak version follows the same route as the SUP, offering paddlers a unique way to explore the scenic waterways and historic cities of Friesland while engaging in a gruelling endurance challenge.

Spanning 220km through the Dutch province of Friesland, the SUP 11-City Tour course passes through 11 historic cities. The challenge lies not only in the distance but also in the conditions. September weather in the Netherlands can be unpredictable, with potential for strong winds and rain, adding to the physical challenge of the race. Participants must navigate narrow canals, open lakes, and under numerous bridges which require skilled paddling. The multi-day format demands consistent performance across several days, testing competitors endurance and recovery.

Participants wishing to enter the kayak category of the SUP 11-City Tour must demonstrate proficiency in long-distance paddling, though specific prior race qualifications are not mandatory. Both solo kayakers and teams can register, with various age and gender categories available. The race encourages a strong community spirit and self-sufficiency, although comprehensive support is provided. Safety gear and adherence to race rules, including the use of appropriate kayaking equipment, are strictly enforced to ensure a safe and enjoyable experience for all.

You can find details about SUP11 City Tour on their official website:
https://sup11citytour.com/

THE CROSSING FOR CYSTIC FIBROSIS

- **Location**.................................... Florida (United States)
- **Time of year**............................ June
- **Approximate distance**................ 129km (80 miles)
- **Average time to finish**................ 12 – 18 hours
- **Average number of entries**.......... 150 participants
- **Average cost to enter**.................. $1000 – $2000
- **Year it started**............................ 2013
- **Support offered**.......................... Supported

The Crossing For Cystic Fibrosis is an endurance paddle challenge that raises awareness and funds for cystic fibrosis, an inherited disorder that affects the lungs and digestive system. The event was founded in 2013 by Travis Suit, whose daughter was diagnosed with cystic fibrosis. Inspired by the benefits of saltwater for those with the condition, Suit created the Crossing as a way to bring the community together and to support those affected by cystic fibrosis. The event has grown significantly over the years, becoming a major fundraiser for the cause. Participants include stand-up paddleboarders, kayakers, and prone paddlers who take on the 80 mile journey from Bimini in the Bahamas to Lake Worth, Florida, across the open waters of the Gulf Stream.

The course is challenging not only because of the distance but also due to the unpredictable nature of the Gulf Stream. Paddlers must navigate strong currents, changing weather conditions, and the possibility of encountering large marine life. The race typically begins in the early morning hours, with participants paddling through the night and into the next day. The isolation of being far from land in open water adds a psychological challenge, making the Crossing as much a mental test as it is a physical one.

Entry is open to paddlers of all levels, but it is recommended that participants have significant experience with long-distance paddling and open-water conditions. All participants must have an escort boat for safety and navigation, and they must complete a qualifying paddle to demonstrate their readiness for the event.

You can find further details about The Crossing on their official website: https://www.crossingforcysticfibrosis.com/

MOLOKAI 2 OAHU

- **Location**..................................... Hawaii (United States)
- **Time of year**............................... July
- **Approximate distance**................. 52km (32.5 miles)
- **Average time to finish**................. 4 – 6 hours
- **Average number of entries**.......... 200
- **Average cost to enter**................... $350 – $450
- **Year it started**............................. 1997
- **Support offered**........................... Supported

The Molokai 2 Oahu Paddleboard World Championships (M2O) is regarded as one of the most prestigious paddleboard races in the world. Established in 1997, it challenges competitors to cross the Kaiwi Channel, one of the most treacherous ocean channels on the planet, known for its powerful currents and large open ocean swells. The race has grown significantly in stature and participation since its inception, attracting the world's top paddleboard athletes. It is celebrated not only as a test of physical endurance and skill but also as a journey through one of Hawaii's most historic waterways.

The 32 mile race across the Kaiwi Channel is daunting due to the channel's notorious conditions, which include strong winds, powerful currents, and massive swells that can reach up to 30 feet. The channel's depth and the ocean conditions often lead to a phenomenon known as "washing machine water," where waves come from multiple directions. Competitors must be adept at water reading, maintaining balance, and energy management over many hours while navigating a direct yet challenging line from Molokai to Oahu.

To enter the M2O, competitors must submit an application that includes details of their paddling background, previous race results, and ocean water experience, as the race organizers prioritise safety and competence in such extreme conditions. Both SUP and traditional prone paddleboards are allowed, and each entrant must secure their own escort boat and crew, which is mandatory for entry. Safety equipment, including a personal flotation device (PFD) and a GPS tracker, is required for all competitors.

You can find details about Molokai 2 Oahu on their official website:
https://www.molokai2oahu.com/

ROWING

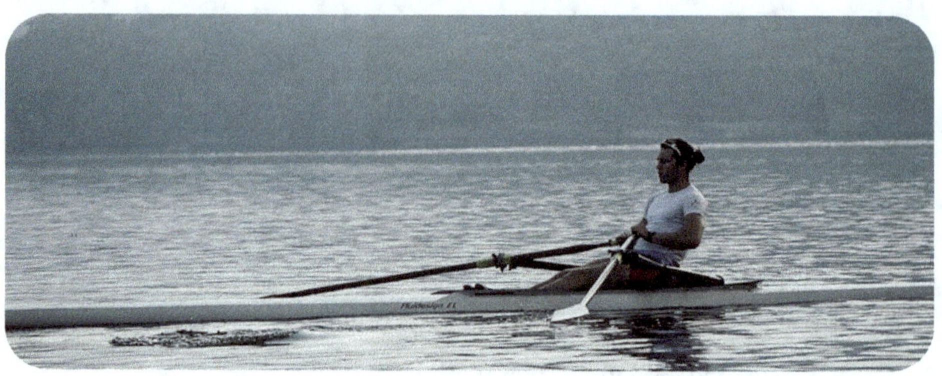

Rowing is a highly competitive sport where athletes propel a boat forward using oars. This sport encompasses various race formats and categories, each demanding specific techniques and strategies. In traditional rowing races, boats are classified by the number of rowers and the type of boat, ranging from single sculls, where one person rows with two oars, to eights, where a crew of eight rowers, each with one oar, works in unison. The primary race formats include sprint races, typically held over distances of 2000 meters on calm water, and head races, which are longer, often ranging from 4000 to 6000 meters, and take place against the clock rather than head-to-head. Rowing races are usually conducted on regatta courses with designated lanes.

Rowing has a rich history that dates back to ancient civilizations, where it was both a means of transportation and a form of competitive sport. The earliest records of rowing come from ancient Egypt, Greece, and Rome, where boats were used for military and ceremonial purposes, and rowing was often depicted in art and literature. In medieval Europe, rowing was primarily associated with commercial and military activities. The modern competitive form of rowing began to develop in the 18th and 19th centuries. The first recorded rowing races were held in England, with the Oxford-Cambridge Boat Race, inaugurated in 1829, becoming a notable event in the sport's history. This race established a tradition of intercollegiate competition that continues today. Rowing gained international prominence with the formation of the International Rowing Federation (FISA) in 1892, which standardized rules and organized world championships. Rowing was introduced to the Olympic Games in 1900 for men and 1976 for women, further cementing its status as a major competitive sport.

The concept of long-distance rowing races has its origins in the early days of the sport, with endurance events evolving as rowing grew in popularity. One of the pioneering long-distance races was the "Head of the River" race, first held on the River Thames in London in 1926.

This annual race, often referred to as the "Head of the River," is a head race format, meaning crews race against the clock over around 4.2 miles. This race, along with similar events such as the "Head of the Charles Regatta" in Boston, which started in 1965, highlighted the endurance aspect of rowing by challenging athletes to maintain speed and technique over longer distances.

Advances in technology have played a significant role in rowing's evolution, with modern rowing boats constructed from lightweight materials such as carbon fibre, allowing for faster speeds and greater efficiency. Training techniques have also become more sophisticated, incorporating sports science, biomechanics, and data analytics to optimize performance and enhance endurance.

The difficulty of a rowing race is influenced by a range of factors, each contributing to the overall challenge of the event. The distance of the race is a fundamental factor, with longer races requiring sustained endurance, strategic pacing, and mental toughness. Water conditions play a crucial role, with rough or choppy water requiring greater skill and adaptability. The synchronization and coordination required in team events, such as eights or fours, add a layer of complexity, as all crew members must work in harmony to achieve optimal performance. Environmental factors, including weather conditions and the presence of other competitors, can also affect the race's difficulty. The physical demands of rowing, including upper body strength, cardiovascular endurance, and technique, are amplified by these elements, making rowing a challenging sport that tests a wide range of athletic abilities.

TALISKER ATLANTIC CHALLENGE

- **Location**..................................... Atlantic Ocean
- **Time of year**............................... December/ January/ February
- **Approximate distance**................. 4828km (3000 miles)
- **Average time to finish**................ 35 – 90 days
- **Average number of entries**.......... 30 – 40 teams
- **Average cost to enter**.................. $20,000 – $30,000
- **Year it started**............................. 1997
- **Support offered**........................... Unsupported

The Talisker Whisky Atlantic Challenge is known as the world's toughest row. It was first held in 1997, inspired by the growing interest in ocean rowing and the challenge of crossing one of the most daunting bodies of water on the planet. Sponsored by Talisker Whisky, this annual race has become a highlight in the extreme sports calendar, attracting competitors from all over the globe. It serves not only as a test of physical endurance but also as a platform for many participants to raise money for charity.

The course covers 3000 miles from the Canary Islands to the Caribbean, making it the premier event in ocean rowing. Rowers face enormous challenges, including fierce ocean storms, towering waves, and the relentless sun. The isolation of the open Atlantic can impose severe psychological strains, from loneliness and fear to sleep deprivation and the monotony of the endless ocean. Additionally, rowers must navigate and maintain their vessel, manage food and water supplies, and deal with any medical emergencies themselves, making it also a profound logistical challenge.

Entry into the Talisker Whisky Atlantic Challenge is open to anyone aged 18 or over, but it requires significant preparation. Participants typically spend 18 months to two years planning and training for the event. This includes passing a series of compulsory courses in sea survival, navigation, and first aid. Teams must also demonstrate their rowing ability, commitment to safety, and physical and mental readiness through a series of assessments and trials.

 You can find details about the Talisker Whiskey Atlantic Row on their website: https://www.worldstoughestrow.com/

GREAT PACIFIC RACE

- **Location**................................... Pacific Ocean
- **Time of year**............................... June
- **Approximate distance**................. 3862km (2400 miles)
- **Average time to finish**................ 30 – 70 days
- **Average number of entries**.......... 10 – 15 teams
- **Average cost to enter**.................. $15,000 – $25,000
- **Year it started**............................ 2014
- **Support offered**.......................... Unsupported

The Great Pacific Race, known as the biggest, baddest human endurance challenge on the planet, offers an unparalleled test of human strength and endurance. Established in 2014, this biennial race has quickly cemented itself as a premier event in ocean rowing, drawing competitive and adventurous rowers from around the world. The race also raises awareness and funds for oceanic environmental issues, emphasizing the need for ocean conservation.

Rowing across the Pacific presents one of the most demanding endurance challenges imaginable. The course stretches over 2,400 miles from the coast of California to Hawaii, taking in some of the most daunting open water conditions on earth, including massive waves, strong winds, and powerful currents. The mental and physical toll of rowing up to 12 hours a day, coupled with the isolation of being at sea for months, adds to the intensity of the challenge.

Entry is a comprehensive process, aimed at ensuring that all participants are fully prepared for the extreme challenges they will face. This includes proving their rowing capability and ocean survival skills through compulsory courses in sea survival, navigation, and first aid. Teams must also procure a specially designed ocean rowing boat equipped with essential safety, navigation, and communication devices. Rigorous inspections of these vessels are conducted to ensure that all equipment meets the safety standards necessary for such an extreme undertaking.

You can find details about Great Pacific Race on their official website:
https://www.worldstoughestrow.com/the-pacific/

GB ROW CHALLENGE

- **Location**... United Kingdom
- **Time of year**............................... June
- **Approximate distance**................. 2900km (1800 miles)
- **Average time to finish**................. 30 – 50 days
- **Average number of entries**.......... 10 – 20 teams
- **Average cost to enter**.................. $10,000 – $15,000 per team
- **Year it started**............................. 2011
- **Support offered**........................... Semi-supported

The GB Row Challenge is a rowing challenge that has captured the imagination of adventurers and rowers alike. Established in 2011, this challenge was inspired by the historical tradition of long-distance rowing and aims to challenge participants with an extreme test of endurance. The race takes place around Great Britain and has quickly gained a reputation as one of the most formidable rowing challenges in the world.

The GB Row Challenge involves an arduous circumnavigation of Great Britain, including a mix of open sea rowing, river navigation, and canal passages, exposing participants to a variety of challenging conditions. Rowers must contend with the unpredictable British weather, including strong winds, rough seas, and changing tides, which can significantly impact their progress and safety.

To enter the GB Row Challenge, participants must meet specific entry criteria to ensure they are prepared for the extreme demands of the race. Teams must include members who are proficient in handling the complex logistics of open sea rowing, including managing tides, weather conditions, and navigation. While individual entries are not generally accepted, teams can consist of varying numbers of rowers, depending on the category chosen. Entry into the race is managed through the official GB Row Challenge website, where teams must submit an application detailing their experience, vessel specifications, and preparedness.

You can find details about the GB Row Challenge on their official website:
https://www.gbrowchallenge.com/

TOUR DU LÉMAN À L'AVIRON

- **Location**.. Switzerland
- **Time of year**................................ September
- **Approximate distance**.................. 160km (99 miles)
- **Average time to finish**.................. 13 – 20 hours
- **Average number of entries**........... 20 – 30 teams
- **Average cost to enter**.................... $350 – $650
- **Year it started**.............................. 1972
- **Support offered**............................. Supported

The Tour du Léman à l'Aviron is a prestigious rowing marathon that has been held annually on Lake Geneva since 1972. It is the longest non-stop rowing regatta in Europe, attracting both amateur and professional rowers from around the world. Originally established to challenge the endurance of university rowing teams, the event has grown to include various categories and has become a highlight in the European rowing calendar. It celebrates the rowing traditions of the region and the beauty of Lake Geneva.

The course of the Tour du Léman à l'Aviron encompasses a full circuit of Lake Geneva, starting and finishing in Geneva. This race is challenging due to its length and the variable conditions on the lake. Rowers must contend with potential strong winds, shifting currents, and unpredictable weather, which can turn a flat lake into a demanding test of skill and stamina. Nighttime rowing adds an additional layer of difficulty, requiring teams to navigate in the dark while battling fatigue. The need for constant coordination and efficient stroke technique makes this race a true test of rowing prowess and team dynamics.

The entry into the Tour du Léman à l'Aviron is open to experienced rowers who can handle long-distance rowing challenges. Participants can enter as solo rowers or as part of a crew. All entrants must provide their rowing credentials, and teams are required to have a thorough understanding of marathon rowing tactics and safety procedures. Each boat must be equipped with necessary navigation lights, safety equipment, and communication devices. Crews must also demonstrate their ability to handle their craft under various weather conditions, as safety checks are a mandatory part of the registration process.

You can find info about The Tour du Léman à l'Aviron on their official website: https://bcge.tourduleman.ch/

RINGVAART REGATTA

- **Location**.. Netherlands
- **Time of year**............................... June
- **Approximate distance**................. 100km (62 miles)
- **Average time to finish**................. 8 – 12 hours
- **Average number of entries**.......... 150 – 200 boats
- **Average cost to enter**.................. $50 – $100
- **Year it started**............................ 1976
- **Support offered**........................... Supported

The Ringvaart Regatta is a unique endurance rowing event that has been challenging participants since 1976. Originally conceived by students from the Delft University of Technology as a marathon rowing race to celebrate the university's 134th anniversary, it has evolved into an annual tradition that attracts a wide range of rowers, from competitive university teams to enthusiastic amateurs. The event is celebrated for its community atmosphere and the physical challenge it represents, making it a highlight of the Dutch rowing calendar.

The 100km course is renowned for its length and the endurance required to complete it. Starting in Leiden, participants row through the Ringvaart canal, encircling the entire Haarlemmermeer polder before finishing in Delft. Navigational skills are tested as rowers must manage long, straight stretches of water, which can become monotonous and physically draining. Additionally, the weather can significantly affect the race, with wind and rain often complicating conditions and testing the crews' abilities to maintain pace and direction over many hours.

Entry into the Ringvaart Regatta is open to a variety of rowing boats, including singles, doubles, fours, and eights. Participants range from experienced rowers to those new to long distance events. Each team or solo rower must demonstrate the capability to handle the physical demands of the distance, and all participants are required to follow strict safety regulations. Prior long-distance rowing experience, while not compulsory, is highly recommended due to the gruelling nature of the race.

You can find details about the Ringvaart Regatta on their official website:
https://ringvaartregatta.nl/

CONCLUSION

As we come to the end of The World's Toughest Endurance Races, I hope you've found inspiration, motivation, and perhaps a new challenge that sparks your interest. As I said in the introduction, covering 150 races across 20 different sports, this book is not just a collection of tough events, it's a testament to the resilience of the human endeavours, the desire to push boundaries, and the incredible feats we are capable of when we embrace discomfort and set out to test our limits.

From ultra-marathons, Ironman triathlons to sailing across oceans, these races represent far more than physical endurance. They are a blend of mental toughness, strategy, and the ability to adapt to nature's harshest environments. Each race carries with it a unique story of struggle and perseverance. The athletes who tackle these challenges are united by a shared mindset, the pursuit of seeing just how far the body and mind can be pushed.

While some of these races may seem extreme or even impossible, they remind us that endurance isn't just about the miles, the climbs, or the time on the clock, it's about the journey, the commitment to growth, and the personal transformation that comes with taking on such monumental challenges. Whether you're an experienced athlete or someone considering your first endurance race, there's something in these pages for you.

Endurance racing is constantly evolving, with new events emerging, distances stretching, and limits being redefined. The community that surrounds these races is growing, and the spirit of adventure that drives it is stronger than ever. My hope is that this book not only introduces you to some of the toughest races on the planet but also encourages you to set your own goals, take on your own challenges, and explore the boundaries of what you thought was possible.

So, as you close these pages, I leave you with one question, what will your next race be? Now it's your turn to lace up, dive in, or saddle up. See you at the starting line.

Thanks for reading.

Jack

AUTHOR

Jack Harrison is a helicopter engineer, ultra-endurance athlete, and avid traveller who has explored over 80 countries. His passion for sport and adventure began at a young age, starting with football. However, Jack soon realized that individual sports aligned more with his desire for accountability and personal achievement. It was triathlon, which was gaining popularity at the time, that truly ignited his love for endurance sports.

By 16, Jack had already earned sponsorships and was placing highly in regional and national competitions. His athletic success was matched by professional experience in property development, but by the age of 25, Jack's focus shifted from competition to testing his mental and physical limits. Over the years, he has taken on some of the world's most gruelling endurance challenges, including Ironman races, long-distance swims, ultra-marathons, sailing across seas, and summiting some of the world's highest mountains.

With over 15 years of experience as a high-level athlete across more than 15 sporting disciplines, Jack continues to push boundaries. Today, he travels the world coaching and instructing various sports, as well as providing strength and conditioning and exercise rehabilitation services. Despite his packed schedule, his passion for endurance racing remains undiminished. Whenever the words "challenge" or "race" are mentioned, Jack's enthusiasm is evident, he's always ready for the next competition or adventure.

His unique blend of professional expertise and extensive athletic experience offers a rare perspective on endurance and the limits of human potential.

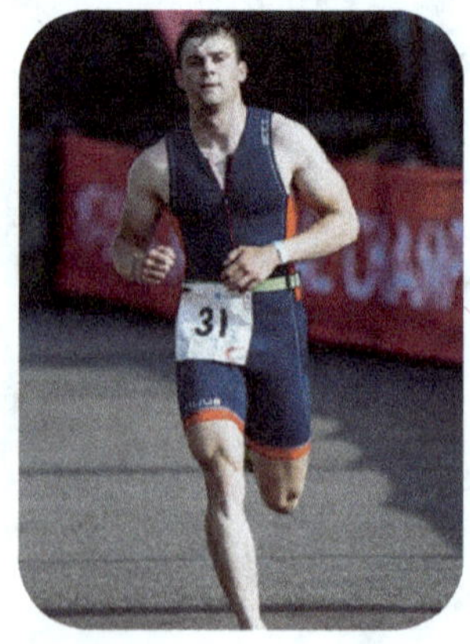